What Doctors Are

"It is a delight to read a comprehensive overview of circumcision unfettered by emotional testimonials and zealous diatribe. There is no one more knowledgeable regarding the topic than Dr. Edgar Schoen. Sgt. Joe Friday of Dragnet fame would be pleased with what is contained within this tome . . . 'Just the facts, ma'am'!"

—Tom Wiswell, MD
Neonatologist and Medical Researcher

"An honest, informative review of circumcision by one of the world's leading authorities that will help anyone who is open-minded wade through the sea of disinformation available to reach the truth."

—Samuel A. Kunin, MD, FACS.
Board Certified Urologist and author of
Circumcision, Its Place in Judaism, Past and Present

"Dr. Edgar Schoen is one of the foremost authorities on all aspects of circumcision in the world and his new book is a fair, honest and insightful account of the extensive health benefits of this simple procedure. This subject has conjured up extremist sentiment, having a detrimental impact on public health and individual well-being. It is so good to have an authoritative book like this to turn."

—Dr. Brian J. Morris
Professor of Molecular Medical Sciences
School of Medical Sciences
University of Sydney

"Dr. Schoen does a terrific job of telling the 'Circumcision Story' from a fresh perspective. The story and the information will be of great use to those of us practicing down in the trenches of today's medicine. The parents of our little patients will find it most useful."

—Thomas Snyder, Urologist
Retired Chief of Urology, Kaiser Medical Center, Martinez CA

"This well researched book presents the scientific evidence supporting the medical benefits of circumcision. It is a valuable resource for policy makers and health care practitioners."

—Myles B. Abbott, MD

"By avoiding medical jargon and obscure technical terms, Dr. Schoen has provided parents with a highly readable summary of the evidence concerning the benefits and risks of neonatal circumcision. I recommend it to any expecting parent or family physician."

—Robert C. Bailey, PhD, MPH
Professor of Epidemiology, School of Public Health
University of Illinois at Chicago

"As a practicing adult/pediatric urologist and Mohel in the san Francisco Bay area, I applaud and appreciate my colleague's efforts to educate and enlighten those that are willing to listen and learn. His honest approach to this controversial issue is refreshing. Dr. Schoen provides a valuable resource for parents and anyone interested in learning the truth about circumcision.

—Joel A. Piser, MD
Berkeley, California

1/12/08

Bob – Best wishes for 2008.

Ed Schoen

Ed Schoen, MD

on

CIRCUMCISION

Timely Information for

Parents and Professionals

from America's #1 Expert

on Circumcision

RDR Books
Berkeley, California

Ed Schoen, MD on Circumcision

RDR Books
2415 Woolsey Street
Berkeley, CA 94705
Phone: (510) 595-0595
Fax: (510) 228-0300
E-mail: read@rdrbooks.com
Website: www.rdrbooks.com

ISBN: 1-157143-123-3

Library of Congress Catalog Card Number 2005902152

Design and Production: Richard Harris
Proofreading: Dianne Yeakey

Distributed in Canada by Starbooks Distribution,
100 Armstrong Way, Georgetown, ON L7G 5S4

Distributed in the United Kingdom and Europe by
Roundhouse Publishing Ltd., Millstone, Limers Lane,
Northam, North Devon EX39 2RG, United Kingdom

Printed in Canada

Acknowledgements

I am grateful to the medical pioneers of the late 19th and early 20th centuries. Their astute clinical observations lead to the acceptance of newborn circumcision as the standard of care for United States males, and set the stage for future confirmatory research studies.. These physicians include Drs. Lewis Sayre, Peter Remondino, J. Henry Simes, Norman H. Chapman, J. M. McGee, and the British physician Oliver H. Fowler. They saw the big picture, recognizing the multiple lifetime benefits of newborn circumcision in preventive health care and cleanliness. They also were fortunate in having the trust, loyalty and confidence of the population they served. The American public was and is independent, open to change, willing to be convinced by facts and to break with tradition. There was no organized resistance to the acceptance of circumcision in contrast to the anti-circumcision activists of today.

By the turn of the 21st century a new group of physicians and scientists have used both laboratory and clinical research to provide convincing evidence of the medical benefits of newborn circumcision in preventing a variety of medical disorders. The new breed of scientists differs from their 19th century colleagues by the nature of their observations which are more objective and specialized. Although many researchers have contributed to the evidence I feel that special mention should go to the following medical professionals and

scientists for their work over the past decades: Abraham
Wolbarst and Archie Dean (penile cancer), Thomas Wiswell
(infant kidney infections), X. Castellsague (cervical cancer),
D.W.Cameron, F.A.Plummer, J. C. and P. Caldwell, Stephen
Moses, Daniel Halperin, Robert Bailey, Roger Short (HIV
and other sexually transmitted diseases).

Special thanks to Stefan Bailis who has intensively reviewed the myriad of publications on circumcision and has
been a gracious and invaluable source of information. Brian
Morris has also been very helpful as a resource. Trinh To has
provided valuable technical assistance.

Finally, I am grateful to my family. My wife Fritzi and our
children, Melissa and Eric, along with their spouses Andy
and Amy have been encouraging and helpful, even when they
would have preferred talking about other topics. I cherish
their assistance and support. My wife's affection, insight, in-
telligence, logic and common sense have kept me on the right
track.

Contents

Preface

In 1987 my best friend Dr Martin Shearn, a noted rheumatologist, was not encouraging when I told him that I accepted the Chairmanship of the Task Force on Circumcision of the American Academy of Pediatrics. At the time, he was Chief of Medicine at Kaiser Permanente, a large Health Maintenance Organization (HMO) in Oakland, California, and I was Chief of Pediatrics. Basically what Marty said was, "Ed, you have had a long and productive career in pediatrics and pediatric endocrinology. You don't need this. Just the mention of circumcision stirs up a hornet's nest, and you could be the one stung." Dr. Shearn pointed out that I would be dealing with not just medical evidence and scientific evaluation, but with highly emotional, biased, activist lay anti-circumcision groups, skilled at gaining media attention for their "cause," the elimination of newborn circumcision. If the Task Force conclusions did not agree with their strong convictions I would be in for trouble. I would be dealing with non-professionals with an agenda and an attitude. Further, he noted, it wouldn't enhance my career, since circumcision is not exactly a prestigious field of scientific study. Some do not consider it to be a bona fide medical procedure, but only of cultural and religious interest. Physicians receive very little education or practical training concerning circumcision, either in medical school or in practice. Marty told me that I might end up being remembered as "Dr. Circumcision" as my medical legacy. He suggested that, as a pediatric endocrinologist, I would be much better off professionally and personally if I continued to devote my efforts to my other medical interests.

But I thought that I could maintain my current pediatric responsibilities, and at the same time head up an evidence-based investigation into the studies that could help clarify the medical validity, if any, of newborn circumcision. I shouldn't have been so naïve. It's true that objective assessments of the data, documentation, and research studies on circumcision were straightforward and would not have detracted much from my other professional interests. What I didn't count on was the determination, organization, persistence, and degree of activism and media influence of the organized anti-circumcision forces. Even before our first Task Force meeting I had received numerous opinions, anecdotes and testimonials, almost all from opponents of circumcision. The print, radio and television media were deluged. Talk shows were replete with advocates preaching in favor of the "intact" state of the male genitals.

When we released our report in 1989 reversing the previous anti-circumcision stance of the AAP by listing medical advantages as well as disadvantages of newborn circumcision there was an outcry from the opposition groups. I was surprised at this reaction, since our conclusions were very moderate, and we didn't make a recommendation for or against circumcision. We simply cited the evidence of the benefits and risks and left the decision up to the parents. There were proven advantages of newborn circumcision, including the virtual elimination of cancer of the penis later in life, prevention of the complications of tight foreskin and local infection, and ease of genital hygiene. Disadvantages were pain, and the possibility of surgical complications, including infection and bleeding. We felt that at the time there was not sufficient data to confirm the protective effect of circumcision against infant kidney infection, cervical cancer. or HIV/AIDS (since then this evidence has become conclusive).

During the following decade, from 1989-1999, I was asked by the AAP to respond to the reactions of the public, the medical profession and the media on matters concerning newborn circumcision as the representative of the AAP. I was quoted in the press, and appeared on talk radio and television programs, often in opposition to anti-circumcision leaders. Sadly, Marty Shearn is no longer here to see the truth of his predictions, but I (along with Dr. Tom Wiswell, the discoverer of the protective effect of circumcision against infant kidney infections) have become the focus of the wrath of the anti's. On a personal level, relationships with opponents of circumcision have varied from friendly discussions to physical threats against me.

But there are positives that have made my involvement with the circumcision issue satisfying and stimulating. I have become familiar with dedicated researchers who are willing to undertake scientific studies in this controversial field. I have been able to perform and publish my own research on penile cancer and infant kidney infections, using data from the large Kaiser Permanente Health Plan population. Above all, I have gained respect for the wisdom of the American public, which has continued to choose circumcision for the great majority of newborn boys, and which has been far ahead of the biased opinions of the organized anti-circumcision groups as well as the disinterest and misleading pronouncements of medical professional organizations, particularly the American Academy of Pediatrics. In this book I believe that parents will find the scientific evidence which validates their choice in favor of newborn circumcision.

Edgar J. Schoen, M.D.
Dec 2004

Introduction and Overview

"Circumcision is like a substantial and well-secured life annuity; every year of life you draw the benefits. Parents cannot make a better paying investment for their little boys." These words were written more than a century ago by Dr. P.C. Remondino, a prominent California physician, in a landmark 1891 book titled *History of Circumcision: Moral and Physical Reasons for Its Performance.* This classic review, which went through 2 printings at the turn of the 20th century, established Remondino as one of the pioneers in the era of modern circumcision in the United States because it was the first publication to analyze and document the medical reasons for infant circumcision. Circumcision had an important historic role beginning with the ancient Egyptians and the Old Testament Hebrews. Among those whose lives have been changed by circumcision are the patriarch Abraham, King Louis XVI of France and Marie Antoinette, Eva Peron, the artist Diego Rivera, and Prince Charles and his 2 sons. In the Judeo-Christian world, a covenant between Abraham and God established that all male infants would be circumcised at age 8 days (Genesis, Chapter 17), and Jesus, being a Jew, was circumcised accordingly (Luke, Chapter 2, Verse 21). Circumcision also has a strong tradition in Islam. Mohammed the Prophet was circumcised, and Abraham is recognized as a patriarch by Muslims.

Remondino knew that in infancy and childhood uncircumcised boys had difficulties with foreskin retraction and cleaning which could lead to local infection. In an era when cleanliness was next to godliness, young parents took the hygiene issue seriously. By the early 1900's middle and upper class families began having their infants circumcised. Cultural and religious groups practicing circumcision were known to have less chance of getting certain sexually transmitted diseases (STDs), particularly syphilis, a scourge in pre-antibiotic times equivalent to AIDS today. In addition, there was evidence that genital cancer was more common when a foreskin was present, including cancer of the penis in older men and cervical cancer in women with uncircumcised male sexual partners.

Let us fast forward to 1987 when I received a call from the American Academy of Pediatrics (AAP) asking me to chair a six-member Task Force on Circumcision. The AAP wanted to analyze and respond to a large study from the Walter Reed Army Medical Center, which found that newborn circumcision prevented severe urinary tract infections (UTIs) in baby boys under the age of 1 year. If true, this finding could overturn the 1971 anti-circumcision position of the AAP. The Army study showed a protective effect of newborn circumcision against severe infant kidney infections. The investigator, Lt. Col. Thomas Wiswell, the Director of Newborn Services at Walter Reed, had been opposed to newborn circumcision. To his surprise, his research on 200,000 newborns found that UTIs were 10-20 times more common in uncircumcised boys and occurred in about 1% of all such infants. These results converted Wiswell from a doubter into a believer in newborn circumcision. In my case, as Chief of Pediatrics at a large HMO, I was involved in teaching, as well as practice, and was aware of Wiswell's work, but felt that it needed confirmation, and I agreed to chair the AAP Circumcision Task

Force. Our charge was to look at other benefits and risks of newborn circumcision, as well as UTIs. I was encouraged that the six-member group would be broad-based and represent the full AAP and not just the viewpoint of neonatologists (newborn specialists), the group responsible for the anti-circumcision AAP statements in 1971 and 1975. The report of our Task Force, issued in 1989, changed the position of the AAP from anti-circumcision to a neutral stance. The report stated that there were both advantages and disadvantages of newborn circumcision, but made no recommendations for or against the procedure. It was felt that Wiswell's evidence of the protection of circumcision against UTIs was suggestive, but needed confirmation by other studies. The reports from Africa indicating that circumcised men were less likely to contact human immunodeficiency virus (HIV) when exposed to infected women, were felt to be important, but too preliminary to be convincing at that time.

In the decade from 1989-1999, proof favoring newborn circumcision continued to mount. At least nine other studies confirmed Wiswell's work showing a greatly increased risk of UTI in uncircumcised baby boys. In Africa, where AIDS has become an epidemic with over 20 million deaths, more than 20 separate studies showed that circumcision offered protection; uncircumcised men were from 3 to 7 times more likely to get infected with HIV after heterosexual exposure than were circumcised men. Further, the issue of pain had been addressed. Local anesthesia was found to be both safe and effective in newborns. With added convincing evidence of the health benefits of circumcision and reassurance on the relief of pain, the arguments in favor of circumcision seemed more valid, and it appeared time to reassess the position of the AAP. In 1999, a new Task Force on Circumcision was formed, which seems, in retrospect, to have been strongly influenced by anti-circumcision forces within and outside of the AAP. Compelling and proven evidence of benefits were referred to as "potential benefits," and these advantages were not considered "sufficient" to recommend routine newborn circumcision. There was no hint as to how much proof would be sufficient to satisfy the 1999 Task Force. Lay anti-circumcision jargon was used (circumcision was referred to as "amputation"). Understandably, the media interpreted the 1999 AAP report's position on circumcision as a step backward, although the body of the report itself documented 6 preventive health benefits, and only one proven disadvantage. This sole risk was that of post operative complications (infection and bleeding), which were said to be "rare and usually mild." The medical evidence and references contained in the report itself belied the misleading negative conclusions. To describe the 1999 AAP report as a "cover-up" might be too strong a statement, but never underestimate the determination of an organization to justify an earlier erroneous policy.

Between 1999 and the present, evidence has continued to accumulate confirming the lifelong disease protection of newborn circumcision. Further proof has been found on the preventive effect of circumcision against UTIs in infancy and penile cancer in older men. Studies in leading medical journals have debunked the myth of improved sexual satisfaction in uncircumcised men. The U.S. Agency for International Development (USAID) has issued a report documenting findings from underdeveloped countries, mainly in Africa, of the decreased prevalence of HIV/AIDS in circumcised men. Adult circumcision is being advised by some to help prevent HIV until a vaccine or completely effective treatment is available. Cervical cancer, the second most common cancer in women, has been shown to be a sexually transmitted disease, and is caused by a virus (human papilloma virus) which is 3 times more common in uncircumcised than in circumcised men. In the face of this additional compelling information favoring circumcision, there has been no comment from the AAP. Medical practitioners who have gotten little information about circumcision during their training, have largely steered away from advising parents on this emotional issue. Much of the circumcision counseling has been pre-empted by the lay anti-circumcision groups, which dominate the media and the Internet.

In modern medical terms, newborn circumcision is analogous to infant immunizations because it is a pediatric health measure, which prevents future disease. Medical evidence shows that the benefits of circumcision accrue over a lifetime, while the adverse effects are immediate and usually minor. The long-term pluses far outweigh the short-term minuses. That's how immunizations work. However, a difference exists between the protective effects of circumcision and those of vaccines. With conventional immunization, 1 vaccine prevents 1 disease. In the case of circumcision one simple, safe procedure has multiple future benefits, extending over a lifetime.

Our primary goal is to present evidence to parents, so they can make an informed decision on circumcision for their newborn son. Based on the medical evidence I favor newborn circumcision, but parents must make their own choice. I have tried to avoid medical jargon and technical terms, and have included references for those parents and practitioners who want to go to the sources and examine the scientific facts further. This book is divided into 2 major sections, called Part I, Proof (Chapters 1-10), which is concerned with medical evidence, and Part II, Consequences (Chapters 11-15), which concentrates on the subjective and emotional factors, and the responses of the public and health professionals. Those readers interested only in the facts and data can stop reading after Part I (Chapter 10). Part II adds the spice.

Prologue

Answers Are Needed.
What Are the Questions?

Although the great majority of American males, over 100 million, have been circumcised, the procedure is still controversial. There is a good deal of confusion among the public as well as among medical providers about the benefits of newborn circumcision. In addressing the issue it may be helpful to consider frequently asked questions and documented evidence cited in the following chapters.

Question 1
Question (Q): Are there medical benefits of newborn circumcision?
Answer (A): Yes, there are at least 6 medically proven circumcision advantages, beginning in newborns and continuing through old age. Also important is genital cleanliness, which is most difficult to maintain in infants and elderly who cannot care for themselves.
Documentation (D): Chapters 3-10 and Reference section.

Question 2
Q: Why circumcise helpless newborns rather than waiting until they are older?
A: Foreskin-associated diseases, including kidney infections and local penile problems, begin in the newborn period, and early circumcision offers maximum preventive health benefits. Also the procedure is most easily done in newborns,

who heal quickly and are uniquely adapted to handle stress.
D: Chapters 1-4, 12 and Reference section.

Question 3
Q: Why is non-religious circumcision widely performed in the United States and not in the rest of the world?
A: For over 100 years Americans have been convinced of the health and hygiene benefits of circumcision, and their wisdom has been confirmed by continuing medical evidence.
D: Chapters 2, 13, 14 and Reference section.

Question 4
Q: Aren't parents robbing infants of their civil rights by agreeing to newborn circumcision? Shouldn't they wait until they are old enough to make the decision for themselves?
A: Nonsense. Parents have not only the moral and legal right but the responsibility to consent to a medical procedure with proven preventive health benefits, whether it is circumcision or immunizations.
D: Chapters 1, 2, 11, 12 and Reference section.

Question 5
Q: Isn't sex better with a foreskin?
A: No, and there are cases where it is worse. Over the past decade there have been multiple studies that show no significant differences between circumcised and uncircumcised men regarding sexual activity and pleasure. And there is evidence that women prefer the circumcised penis, mainly for reasons of hygiene.
D: Chapters 9, 11 and Reference section.

Question 6
Q: What are the complications of newborn circumcision?
A: When properly performed by an experienced operator cir-

cumcision is quick and safe. But it is an operation. According to the American Academy of Pediatrics the complications of newborn circumcision are rare and usually minor, with about 1 in 300 having mild infection or bleeding. Serious injury or death are extremely rare and are usually caused by surgical negligence or the inappropriate use of general anesthesia
D: Chapters 1, 2 and Reference Section.

Question 7
Q: My son is 6 years old and we didn't have him circumcised as an infant. I feel we made a mistake. Should we have him circumcised now?
A: That is a more difficult question than newborn circumcision. Circumcision at this age is more complicated and expensive and experienced operators are not as easy to find. But there are still many future benefits, and the decision by the parents should be based on both social and medical factors.
D: Chapters 2, 4, 5-10 and Reference section.

Question 8
Q: What should be done about the pain of circumcision?
A: Newborns feel pain just like everyone else and local anesthesia should be given for all circumcisions. Although a nerve block is usually used (as with dental anesthesia), there is also an anesthetic cream. General anesthesia should never be used for infant circumcision.
D: Chapter 2 and Reference section.

Question 9
Q: The foreskin is normal body tissue. Doesn't it have a function?
A: Yes it does, but the role of the foreskin is in the fetus. If the foreskin isn't present during pregnancy the penis doesn't develop normally. But after birth it no longer has a role, and

is a health and hygiene liability. This time-specific function of body tissues is not unusual. The ovaries and uterus are essential for normal female development and childbirth, but after the menopause they are no longer necessary and present a health risk.

D: Chapter 1 and Reference section.

Question 10

Q: What is the best method for performing newborn circumcision?

A: There are three devices used for newborn circumcision; the Mogen clamp, the Gomco clamp and the Plastibell. They all work fine in experienced hands. The parents should concentrate on making sure that whoever performs the procedure has done many circumcisions, and uses some form of local anesthesia.

D: Chapters 1, 2 and Reference section.

PART I – PROOF

1

Why Newborns?
The Window of Opportunity

A newborn baby is a delicate, helpless creature who is ill-suited to cope with the dangers of the outside world. Right? Wrong. Immediately after birth, a full-term infant is tough, adaptable, and resilient. In changing from the dependent fetal state to independent life, the newborn has embarked on the most dangerous journey he will every take. All critical body functions had depended upon a lifeline to the mother and, suddenly, this bond is cut, and he is on his own. He was squeezed through an unforgiving, narrow channel, which could shut down at any time and suffocate him. The dangers of a normal birth make the travails of Indiana Jones look insignificant. But the newborn is ready. All his vital systems—heart, lungs, and brain—are prepared for stress. He is programmed for "fight or flight." The pituitary, or master gland, is primed to release hormones which control strength, energy, and the key body functions. The elevation of the adrenal hormones, adrenaline and hydrocortisone, quickly provide stronger heart contractions and sugar for energy. To keep the newborn baby warm and raise the heart beat, the thyroid hormones reach levels that would only be seen with an overactive gland in older children or adults. There is an outpouring of sex hormones as well. It's as if a normal newborn boy is on steroids. Testosterone, the male hormone, can reach adult levels before it falls to the childhood range.

13

The brain and entire nervous system are also alerted to environmental threats. Outside stimuli, such as pain, hunger, cold, and loud noises, have an instantaneous effect. The baby screams, tightens his muscles, grasps and jerks in a desperate call for help. If relief arrives, usually in the form of parental assistance, calm quickly returns, and all is forgiven and forgotten. There is no time to hold a grudge. Nothing is permanent. Preparation must be made for the next crisis, which will surely happen when the next feeding is due. One cannot dwell on the last traumatic event when it is critical to be ready for the next. If adults responded to hunger like a newborn, restaurants would be filled with a screaming, flailing, red-faced mob at lunchtime. There is no evidence to support claims that painful events in the newborn period are imprinted on the brain and leave a permanent mark. Anti-circumcision groups play a cruel hoax by stating, usually on talk shows or on the Internet that young parents have caused permanent emotional damage to their infant by agreeing to newborn circumcision. The unsupported claims of the circumcision opponents do not always go unchallenged, even in the media. Dr. Phil, the TV psychologist, was faced with the concerns of a new mother who was convinced by anti-circumcision groups that she had done irreparable psychological damage to her infant son by having him circumcised. Dr. Phil minced no words in his reply. He reiterated that the claims of emotional damage by newborn circumcision have no basis in fact, and "are a lot of crap." Amen.

After five decades of pediatric practice, I am still awed by the strength and resilience of babies and their ability to handle major crises, including life-threatening diseases and multiple surgeries. The key to the psychological outcome is not the severity of the trauma, but the response of the parents. Even if an infant has had severe trauma or a major operation, let alone a brief surgical procedure such as circumcision, a loving, attentive family will prevent any long term effects. On the other hand parental insecurity, inadequacy and neglect, and above all, repeated failure to display affection, can lead to later emotional and behavioral problems in the child in the absence of any newborn trauma or disease.

The younger you are, the quicker you heal. and that starts at birth. Broken bones, cuts, and surgical incisions heal faster in babies than in children, and faster in children than in adults. A hernia repair in a newborn is often done without stitches (an adherent substance is applied), and the scar becomes quickly invisible. A 3-year-old is racing around 3 or 4 days after an appendectomy, while it takes an adult weeks to get back to normal after the same operation.

When newborn circumcision is done in the standard fashion (Plastibell, Mogen, or Gomco clamps), no stitches or adherents are necessary. The thin inner and outer parts of the foreskin simply adhere to each other and heal within a week. Within a few hours or even minutes, the baby is acting and feeding normally. If circumcision is postponed to later in infancy or childhood, stitches are needed to bind the foreskin layers, and the convalescent period is extended to a week or longer. A toddler or young child is more vulnerable to the emotional effects than is a newborn, and his bodily defense mechanisms are not as quick to respond. In adults, circumcision is more difficult and takes longer, and healing is slower.

Endorphins, pain relieving hormones produced at the base of the brain, are most effective in the newborn period. Endorphins are secreted in response to exercise, pain and other stressful events. They act on the same sites in the brain as do morphine and other opiates, and are responsible for effects such as a "runner's high" after a long distance event and ignoring a painful injury during an athletic event. It is much easier to stimulate secretion of endorphins in newborns than it is later in life. For example, simply having the baby drink a sugar solution will cause a rise in endorphins and relief of pain, while no such effect is seen in older infants and children, or in adults. This unique ability of the newborn to respond to pain, combined with the proven efficacy and safety of local anesthesia, means that newborn circumcision, properly performed, should be a painless procedure.

How long does this window of opportunity stay open? Up to about the age of two months, if a parent can find a physician willing to perform the procedure after the newborn is discharged from the hospital. Most professionals are not willing to do it in the office. Traditional Jews are circumcised at age 8 days by a "mohel" who is usually a non-physician, often a rabbi or cantor, trained to do the procedure according to religious requirements. Recently, a number of Jewish physicians have qualified religiously as mohels, so they offer double satisfaction to Jewish families, medical ability and traditional values A few physicians, like urologist Dr. Samuel Kunin, will perform non-religious circumcision at any time during the first few months of life, but this is unusual. One problem is that as the infant ages the foreskin thickens, and by the time the baby weighs about 15 pounds, the foreskin layers usually will no longer adhere to each other, as they do in the immediate newborn period, and sutures become necessary.

Circumcision performed after the newborn period is more difficult and traumatic, there are fewer qualified operators, and some of these routinely use general anesthesia, increasing the risk. Complications are more common and healing is slower at older ages, and post-neonatal circumcision is about 10 times as expensive as in newborns.

Thus, the newborn period is the window of opportunity to gain the maximum protective effect of circumcision against disorders ranging from severe infant kidney infections, which are most prevalent within the first few months of life, to penile cancer in middle and old age, with multiple disorders in between, including sexually transmitted diseases, particularly HIV/AIDS. These lifetime advantages will be documented in later chapters. The benefits can be accomplished with minimal and temporary physical and emotional discomfort due to the unique strengths, resilience, and healing powers of newborns, when circumcision is performed within the first few weeks of life.

2

What Is Circumcision?
Why Do It?
How To Do It and What Can Go Wrong?

Newborn circumcision is a minor surgical procedure consisting of removing the small piece of skin covering the head of the penis. The name comes from the Greek, meaning to cut around. In the hands of a skilled operator, it takes only a few minutes and is very safe, but it is an operation and can have complications.

Why remove the foreskin? Doesn't it have a function? After all it is normal body tissue. The reasons for circumcision are lifetime disease prevention beginning at birth, as will be described (Chapters 3-8). Many parents choose circumcision because of ease of genital cleanliness. Yes, the foreskin does have an important function. But, contrary to popular myth and unsubstantiated anecdotes, it has no significant effect on sexual function (see Chapter 9). The role of the foreskin is in the fetus, where it is essential for the normal development of the penis, starting in the third month of pregnancy. As the penis begins to form from primitive tissues, the skin on the shaft grows faster than the shaft itself and folds over to form a hood. This foreskin hood completely encircles the head of the developing penis and is responsible for the normal formation of the end of the penis, including the urinary opening at the center of the tip. If this large foreskin hood is incomplete, an abnormal condition known as hypospadius develops, in which the urinary opening (urethra) opens on the underside of the penis instead of the tip, and the baby is also born with an abnormal, hooded foreskin. Normal penile development is finished before the seventh month of pregnancy. The foreskin has completed its function before birth. From the newborn period onward the foreskin is a liability, and newborn circumcision creates a lifetime health advantage.

This time-sensitive role of normal body tissue is not unique to the foreskin. Other examples are the uterus and the ovaries. These organs are important in female development and childbearing, but are health risks after the menopause. The role of the prostate is controversial early in life, but it presents the dangers of cancer and urinary blockage in elderly men. Similarly, the appendix is only a source of trouble in humans, but in lower species performs an important intestinal function. So, the argument goes, if we do circumcision at birth, when the foreskin no longer has a role, why not remove the uterus, ovaries, prostate and appendix when their useful time is over? The answer, of course, is location, location, location. Although newborn circumcision is a quick, safe, simple procedure, removing the other organs requires risky major surgery.

Pediatricians, obstetricians, or family practitioners perform most newborn circumcisions. In older infants, children and adults circumcision is usually done by a urologist. Skill and experience are the most important factors to consider when choosing an operator, rather than formal specialty. In giving informed consent for newborn circumcision, the family should question the physician on the number of circumcisions he/she has done, the method used, and whether some form of pain control will be used. Three devices are used in newborns to make circumcisions quick and safe—the Gomco clamp, the Plastibell, and the Mogen clamp. The first two have a bell-shaped protector which is placed between the foreskin and glans to protect the head of the penis as the foreskin is cut free.

In all three techniques (Mogen, Gomco and Plastibell) the foreskin must first be separated from the head of the penis using a blunt instrument. Before the advent of the special clamps the foreskin was simply pulled forward and cut off with a sharp knife. Pressure was then applied to control bleeding. The Mogen clamp method is closest to this early technique, and the clamp holds the inner and outer layers of the foreskin together, controlling bleeding and allowing the 2 layers to stick together as the foreskin is cut off away from the clamp. Because of its simplicity the Mogen method is the quickest, and is favored by Jewish religious circumcisers. I have seen these mohels perform a circumcision in less than a minute using a Mogen clamp. The potential problem with the Mogen clamp is that there is no provision to protect the head of the penis, and in inexperienced hands there is a chance of damaging the penis. If the Mogen clamp is to be used, ask how many circumcisions the operator has done; it is very safe in the hands of a skilled operator. Both the Gomco and Plastibell methods protect the head of the penis with a bell-shaped device, metal in the case of the Gomco and plastic in the Plastibell. The Gomco has been around for years and is favored by many physicians, particularly older practitioners, who have had wide experience and feel confident in using it. It is more cumbersome than the Mogen and Plastibell clamps, and it generally takes somewhat longer to do a circumcision with the Gomco. But not necessarily so. Dr Samuel Kunin of Southern California, a good friend, who is both a urologist and a mohel has done over 7000 circumcisions using a Gomco clamp. I have seen him in action and for efficiency and quickness in performing a painless circumcision he is unrivaled. He uses local anesthesia with a special technique he developed. In the case of the Plastibell, a suture is tied around the plastic bell after it is placed over the head of the penis, the foreskin is cut off, and the infant is sent home with the plastic bell in place and the suture holding the 2 foreskin layers together; the plastic bell falls off in 5-7 days. Although the method chosen depends upon the preference of the operator, I feel that the Plastibell method is simplest and most foolproof, and we train young physicians in this technique. I don't think that the parents should be concerned about the method used, but should rather make sure that the operator has broad experience and has done many circumcisions.

Newborns feel pain, and some form of pain relief should be used. An effective form of local anesthesia, which is currently most popular, is called dorsal penile nerve block (DPNB), and it is often given in association with the baby sucking on a sugar solution. DPNB is analogous to dental anesthesia and consists of injecting lidocaine solution with a fine needle into the base of the penis a few minutes before the circumcision. There has also been success with a special anesthetic lidocaine ointment, but this ointment must be applied to the penis at least an hour in advance, and in my experience is not quite as effective as DPNB. Anesthetic ointment is most often used by non-physician religious circumcisers, since the use of injected anesthesia is limited to medical professionals. The age-old Jewish practice of using a small amount of sweet wine has recently been supported by scientific studies, which show that a sugar (sucrose) solution is effective in pain relief in newborns (in rats as well as in humans).The mechanism of sucrose action is stimulation of the secretion of endorphins by the brain; endorphin is a natural pain killer. Sucrose only stimulates endorphins in newborns, and does not work in older children or adults.

Previous hesitation to use even local anesthesia was based on concerns that possible ill effects were unacceptable in a very low-risk operation. In our 1989 AAP report, we were cautious about the use of local anesthesia, since published data, although encouraging, were limited to a small number of cases. But in the past few years, many thousands of newborn circumcisions have been done using DPNB and other forms of local anesthesia and the safety and efficacy have been proven. Nowadays, newborn circumcision should not be done without some form of local anesthesia, which is often given along with oral sucrose solution, and occasionally with oral medication such as acetaminophen (Tylenol). General anesthesia should never be used in newborn circumcision, and should only be used under special circumstances at older ages. The rare fatalities with circumcision have almost all been due to general anesthesia and not to the surgery itself.

Complications

Newborn circumcision is a quick and simple operation with a very low rate of complications when properly performed. But nothing is foolproof, nothing is idiot-proof. Serious complications of newborn circumcision are extremely rare and are almost always due to inexperience, improper technique or negligence The choice of an experienced operator is essential. An example of negligence is a case that occurred a number of years ago in which the physician used an electric cautery in association with a metal clamp, which should never be done, since electricity and metal don't mix. The resultant burn led to a partial amputation of the penis. There have been cases of damage to the head of the penis when an inexperienced operator was using a Mogen clamp. But these are rare exceptions which can be avoided by proper training and experience.

The estimated rate of side effects is 0.3% (about 1 in 300), and these are generally minor, consisting of bleeding or local infection. Serious effects are rare, as noted in the previous paragraph. In 500,000 circumcisions performed in New York State, there were no deaths or penile amputations. Common sense and proper precautions, as well as good surgical technique, must be emphasized. The infant should be healthy and stable. Circumcision should not be performed if there is a family history of a bleeding disorder (e.g., hemophilia) or if the penis is not properly formed (hypospadius). In repairing hypospadius later on the foreskin may be necessary for skin grafting.

In summary, the foreskin can be thought of as an external appendix, a remnant of earlier times and a potential source of lifetime trouble, which can easily and safely be removed at birth.

3

Infant Kidney Infections

The 5-month-old infant boy had a fever of 105.4°, was irrita-
ble, and a little "jerky," though there had not been a convul-
sion and the baby seemed alert. At 3 a.m. the young, on-call
pediatrician quickly dressed and headed for the Emergency
Department after hanging up the phone. She instructed the
triage nurse to bring the fever down with lukewarm spong-
ing. On the way to Emergency, the physician reviewed the
likely diagnoses and "work-up" she would do. She knew that
many diseases, such as viral illnesses and ear infections, can
cause body temperature to rise to 104° in young infants, but
fever in the 105°+ range often signals a serious life-threatening infection. Although she could rattle off a laundry list
of potentially overwhelming infections, the four commonest
were foremost in her mind: meningitis, pneumonia, sepsis
(blood stream infection) and kidney infection (urinary tract
infection or UTI). When she arrived in the Emergency Department, she was confronted by the distraught young parents, recent Chinese immigrants, and she was grateful that
the staff nurse had arranged to have a Cantonese-speaking
nurse come down from the surgical ward. The infant had
been well until about 12 hours ago when the parents noted
the fever, which seemed to go up and down accompanied by
increasing irritability; the infant refused to feed and vomited
once. No obvious site of infection was found on exam and a

"septic work-up" was started—blood drawn for blood count and culture, spinal tap, chest x-ray, and urine for evidence of infection. A tight, unretractable foreskin was noted on exam (remember, most Asians, Hispanics, and Europeans do not generally practice newborn circumcision), which brought two points to mind. Firstly, serious kidney infections are over 10 times more common in uncircumcised than in circumcised infants, and secondly, one must be more invasive to diagnose a UTI if the infant is uncircumcised. A simple "bagged urine" (a plastic bag placed over the penis) yields a valid specimen in circumcised infants, but since the sticky inner mucous surface of the foreskin is both a magnet and a refuge for bacteria, it is impossible to tell if the bacteria-filled urine from an "intact" penis is coming from the foreskin or the kidneys. One must bypass the foreskin either by introducing a tube up the urethra (a "catheterized specimen") or draw urine through a needle introduced directly into the bladder (a "bladder tap"). The spinal fluid and chest x-rays showed no sign of infection, the blood white cell count was very high, indicating bacterial infection, and the bladder urine was filled with pus cells and bacteria (E. coli, an intestinal organism, the most common cause of kidney infections). The antibiotics chosen were appropriate treatment for E. coli kidney and bloodstream infections, and within 36 hours the fever was gone. The physician was relieved that she had made the diagnosis quickly and started treatment. Since the blood culture later showed that the infection had already entered the bloodstream, a delay could have permitted the bacteria to spread to the spinal fluid, leading to meningitis and the possibility of death or brain damage. When the baby was sent home a week later he had an appointment for kidney function studies in a month, both to make sure that there were no underlying abnormalities of the urinary system and to check for damage done by the infection. During her 5 years of training and experience the physician had seen 4 similar kidney infections in infant boys—none were born with kidney abnormalities and all were uncircumcised.

Until the early 1980s, the high rate of serious kidney infections in uncircumcised infant boys was unrecognized. Then in 1982, researchers at the University of Texas investigating kidney infections in infants made a puzzling observation. They knew that UTIs in adults and older children occurred mainly in females, presumably due to the shorter urethra. But in infants below the age of 1 year, they found that most severe kidney infections were in boys - and 95% of these boys were uncircumcised. The authors were able to observe this large series of uncircumcised infants because their study took place close to the Mexican border and their subjects were largely Hispanics, who are not circumcised on a cultural basis. A young neonatologist (newborn specialist) in the U.S. Army, Dr. Tom Wiswell, didn't believe it. Like most neonatologists, he was opposed to newborn circumcision. As Chief of the Neonatology Service at the Walter Reed Army Hospital he was in a position to challenge the Texas study by using the huge data base of the Armed Forces. Dr. Wiswell looked at 200,000 uncircumcised and circumcised infant boys listed in the Armed Services computers and to his amazement found that UTIs in the first year of life were between 10 and 20 times more common in the uncircumcised group. This discovery not only converted Wiswell from anti to pro circumcision, but set up a flurry of other studies. At the Boston Children's Medical Center, Harvard investigators studied infants coming to the Emergency Department with high fevers requiring "septic work-up." They found 35 infant boys with severe kidney infections. All 35 were uncircumcised, in spite of the fact that most (60%) of the infant males in that population were circumcised.

By 1992 there had been 9 major studies of male infant

UTIs in this country and in Europe. Others since then have confirmed the preponderance of UTIs in uncircumcised infant boys. The average "odds ratio" is about 10. That means that an uncircumcised infant boy has 10 times the chance of getting UTI in the first year of life. Proof that circumcision protects against infant UTIs is overwhelming. A study we performed at Kaiser Permanente in 1996 illustrates this point. That year almost 15,000 babies were born in our health plan, and about 10,000 (67%) were circumcised, leaving about 5000 (33%) uncircumcised. We found that 156 infant boys below the age of 1 year were diagnosed with UTI. Although the great majority of boys (67%) had been circumcised, 134 of the 156 UTIs occurred in the one third of boys that had not been circumcised. This is a ten-fold increased risk due to the presence of the foreskin, just as others found previously. This comes out to be 82 baby boys in our health plan in a 1 year period with infant kidney infections which could have been prevented.

Well, you might say, what's the big deal? Just give a little antibiotics and that's the end of it. Not likely. UTIs in infancy can be dangerous, particularly in the first 3 months of life when 20% of babies get spread of the infection to the blood which can carry the dangerous bacteria to other parts of the body, particularly the brain and spinal membranes where they can cause meningitis. The kidneys are not fully developed at birth and continue to mature for the first 3 years. UTIs during this critical period may cause permanent kidney damage. A urologic researcher named Roberts at Tulane University believes that some cases of unexplained kidney failure later in life could have arisen from undiagnosed UTIs in uncircumcised boys during infancy. It has been found that 38% of babies with UTIs will show evidence of kidney scarring and "reflux" if an imaging study is done 1 year later. Reflux refers to backing up of dye into the kidneys and is associated with kidney damage. A large multinational study by urologists comparing American and European boys (who are rarely circumcised) found reflux to be more common in the Europeans. Also, there is a condition found in some infants at the time of UTI in which the kidneys lose salt and there is a large increase in certain hormones (aldosterone and renin) which are associated with high blood pressure. There are no proven data so far on the long term dangers of infant UTIs. But serious long term damage is certainly a possibility. The kidney is a vital organ, so why subject your baby to the risk when infant UTIs can be almost completely prevented by newborn circumcision?

How does the presence of a foreskin put an infant at risk for UTIs? The proof here is on firm scientific ground. As mentioned, the sticky inner surface of the foreskin is both a magnet and a haven for bacteria, and though urine from a normal circumcised male is sterile, it is contaminated with bacteria if the foreskin is present. We know a lot about the contaminating bacteria. They are normal inhabitants of the intestinal tract, known as E.coli. And not just any E.Coli. The organisms usually causing kidney infections—known as "uropathic" bacteria—are "fimbriated" E. coli, meaning that they have tentacles which act as suction cups in binding to the inner foreskin layers from whence they make their way up to the kidney. A Swedish scientist named Fussel published remarkable photos taken through an electron microscope showing fimbriated E.coli, the UTI culprit, bound closely to the foreskin inner surface, but absent from the skin cells of the head of the penis.

Why were infant UTIs not as commonly diagnosed prior to the 1980s? One reason for the previous lack of recognition is that infantile UTI is a "silent" disease. It cannot be diagnosed by physical examination. You won't find it if you don't look for it by doing a proper sterile urine culture. Perhaps in the past infants with high fever and elevated white blood counts were simply treated with antibiotics without a specific diagnosis. I would like to offer another possibility. Our new, super-efficient, form-fitting plastic diapers might be to blame. Not long ago there was an epidemic in young women of "toxic shock syndrome" with a high fatality rate. This overwhelming infection was found to be due to highly absorptive vaginal tampons which prevented menstrual fluids from properly draining, allowing staphylococcus bacteria to multiply and produce dangerous toxins. Similarly, our new diapers are so efficient that even in the case of diarrhea, there is no leakage, the baby remains clean, and there is less odor. In the days of cloth diapers, smelly diarrheal stools would run down the infant's legs, causing a mess, but now the feces is held tightly inside to be pressed against the uncircumcised penis. The tentacled intestinal bacteria and the magnetic inner foreskin are kept in close contact, which can lead to an infection which ascends up to the kidneys.

To carry the "tight diaper syndrome" reasoning to its logical conclusion suggests a remedy for those favoring the "natural" uncircumcised penis. In primitive, diaperless societies, infants' excrement simply fell to the floor of the cave or jungle or desert. There was no contact between feces and foreskin, diminishing the chance of harmful intestinal bacteria attaching to the foreskin and ascending the urinary tract to cause serious kidney infection. Those parents opposed to circumcision, but wishing to protect their infant boys from urinary infection, could simply forego diapers. This diaperless state would certainly be natural, but it might not be acceptable for practical and esthetic reasons. So it still looks like newborn circumcision is the best bet to avoid serious kidney infections in infant boys. Even if the diaperless state was acceptable and would help prevent infant UTIs, this still would not effect the protection offered by newborn circumcision against HIV/STDs, penile cancer, uterine cancer, and local problems which occur later in life.

It has been shown that in older boys and young men UTIs are more common in those who are uncircumcised, but at these later ages UTIs are milder, less common and have fewer complications. It is in infancy, when they are more prevalent and dangerous, that UTI prevention is most important, and this requires newborn circumcision.

4

Local Penile Problems

The Austrian Empress, Maria Theresa, knew something was seriously wrong within a month after the marriage of her daughter, Marie Antoinette, to King Louis XVI of France. The newlyweds were still teenagers, and both were robust, but their sex life was not clicking. Marie Antoinette's letters home were quite specific. It wasn't that Louis wasn't interested. He seemed raring to go and easily excited, but when the time came for penetration, he was more than just discouraged. He was in pain, and the urge soon disappeared. Responding to the crisis of a potentially sexless, heirless marriage, the Empress Maria arranged for a discrete analysis of the problem. It turned out that the young King Louis was suffering from phimosis, a condition in which the tip of the foreskin is tightly constricted, making it impossible to retract and resulting in painful erections. Sexual intercourse became an ordeal. The cure is circumcision, but understandably, the young king was reluctant, given the surgical and anesthetic deficiencies of the 18th century. Instead, he devoted himself to acceptable macho activities, such as riding, hunting, and drinking, leaving the queen to fend for herself. Finally, after steady diplomatic and royal influence was brought to bear (and internal hormonal pressures as well), King Louis XVI was circumcised at age 22. According to follow-up corre-

spondence between Marie Antoinette and her mother, subsequent sexual performance was fine and the requisite heirs
were produced. But, as you know, the ending was not happy
and through the action of the guillotine, the king later lost a
part of his anatomy more essential than the foreskin, as did
his queen.

Phimosis is present in 0.5-1% of males and is most likely
to become obvious at puberty when penis growth and fre-
quent erections occur, and the glans becomes trapped in the
tight foreskin. Local penile and urinary infection might call
attention to it in infancy or early childhood. Phimosis must
be distinguished from an adherent ("undifferentiated") foreskin. The foreskin is normally bound to the head of the penis
(glans) at birth and gradually separates ("differentiates"),
usually by age 1-3 years. But although the foreskin normally adheres to the glans in infancy and early childhood, the
opening at the end is wide and can be retracted. In phimosis,
the foreskin opening is not much bigger than the size of a
pinhead. Although it permits the escape of urine, it can never
be drawn back over the glans to permit cleansing or allow
for proper penile expansion during erection, even after it has
separated from the glans.

Phimosis can be missed in early infancy because of normal foreskin adherence to the glans. Since circumcision is
the only treatment for true phimosis, this means that surgery
is required later in childhood or adolescence, when the procedure is more complex, traumatic, and expensive, and may
require the added risk of general anesthesia.

In some boys, the opening in the foreskin is not pinpoint,
as in phimosis, but is simply smaller than normal so that
when the foreskin is retracted, it becomes caught behind the
glans and cannot be returned to home base. This tight con-
striction shuts off circulation and the penile head becomes
swollen and painful. Kind of like getting your hand stuck

between metal bars and not being able to pull it out. With quick action and steady pressure on the glans, the foreskin can be popped back into place. In some instances, surgery is necessary. This unhappy state of affairs is known as paraphimosis. I've seen about a dozen cases and luckily have been able to reduce them all nonsurgically.

A combination of tight, adherent foreskin and poor genital hygiene can lead to an unpleasant infection of the foreskin and glans called balanoposthitis. The entire front end of the penis, head and covering, becomes red, swollen, and painful, and there is often a smelly, yellow discharge. Warm soaks and antibiotics relieve the infection, but it can recur, necessitating circumcision. A study in England found that about 4% of uncircumcised boys will at some time develop balanoposthitis, and it is most often seen in boys between the ages of 3 and 5 years.

Penile irritation due to unhygienic conditions and sand under the foreskin in combination with a lack of water for washing, as is the case in desert regions, increase the chances of getting local foreskin infections. This happened to the U.S. Army in World War II in the North African campaign, as will be detailed in Chapter 10.

Constricting and infected foreskins—phimoses, paraphimoses, and balanoposthitis—are unpleasant and painful reminders of the value of newborn circumcision. No foreskin means no phimosis, paraphimosis, or balanoposthitis. Avoidance of significant medical diseases is the great benefit of newborn circumcision in my mind, but the more mundane advantages of everyday cleanliness and ease of maintenance are the practical factors that cause many parents to choose to have their baby circumcised. This was the case with American middle class parents 100 years ago. Then as now parents preferred circumcision for their infants for two simple reasons – cleanliness and better health. No one has elucidated the reasons for choosing newborn circumcision better, in my mind, than the best-selling author, Ann Lamott, in her insightful book, *Operating Instructions*, which describes the experiences of a first-time mother of a little boy. Lamott was somewhat aware of some medical advantages of newborn circumcision (she knew about penile cancer), but the determining factors in her choice in favor of circumcision were hygiene and, to a lesser extent, appearance (esthetics). As she put it, when it came to the infant's penis, the problem was "keeping the damn thing clean, presumably with Q-tips and 409. Who's got the time?" In infancy, the task falls to the parent and, later in childhood, to the boy himself. She knew her friends had trouble even getting their boys to wash their hands, and she figured that foreskin/penile cleansing was a lost cause. Also Lamott prefers the appearance of the circumcised penis. "The uncircumcised ones look sort of marsupial, or like little rodents stuck in garden hoses." These are fighting words for a middle class, creative intellectual in Marin County, California, where a decision in favor of newborn circumcision requires a good deal of courage and risks ostracism. In this trendy, environmentalist community, the "intact" or "natural" state is socially correct and "genital chic." Retaining the foreskin is equivalent to preserving the giant redwoods or saving the whales. Anne Lamott might be pleased to know that medical evidence continues to accumulate supporting her pro-circumcision position on genital hygiene, esthetics, and medical benefits and advantages, including the prevention of cancer and HIV/AIDS.

The hygienic status of uncircumcised British schoolboys, ages 5-6 and 14-15 years, was examined in a private boarding school for middle to upper income students where one would expect that cleanliness would be emphasized. It was found that 80% of the uncircumcised sons of privilege could be classified as having poor genital hygiene. In 60% of the

5-6 year olds and 28% of the 14-15 year olds the foreskin was not fully retractable. If uncircumcised middle and upper class boys in an advanced country can't keep their penises clean and foreskins retracted, the situation in underdeveloped countries is best left to the imagination. It is interesting to note that most of the medical publications describing local foreskin problems come from Europe, where routine circumcision is not practiced, though the medical standards are high. England is widely represented with reports of foreskin difficulties, but also Denmark where a report of almost 10,000 boys, age 6-17 years showed a 4% rate of phimosis and 33% adherent foreskin. Uncircumcised men were found to be more likely to have a variety of skin disorders in a recent British publication, including psoriasis, eczema and local infections.

5

An Ignored Weapon Against HIV/AIDS

The twin African villages were situated within a mile of each other on either side of a valley in Zambia. Lozi and Luvale were similar in size and life styles, but there was one significant difference that prevented them from being identical twins. Sacred circumcision was practiced in Luvale while the Lozi were left uncircumcised. Then in the early 1980's tragedy struck in the form of the HIV/AIDS epidemic and it soon became obvious to the villagers themselves that there were many more cases among the uncircumcised men in Lozi. Subsequent testing showed that 20% of young Lozi adults were HIV-positive, while in the nearby Luvale village the rate was 7%, 3 times lower. It was calculated that if the epidemic continued at the same rate 60% of the Lozi children would die of AIDS. The Lozi parents recognized this danger, and in defiance of tradition and the village elders, began to take their young sons to other villages to be circumcised.

At about the same time, in 1985, an anthropologist named Priscilla Reining, was working with the Haya tribe in Tanzania near Lake Victoria, and she wondered why the Hayas were getting more AIDS than other tribes in the region. She concluded that the high rate of AIDS was related to the fact that circumcision was not practiced by the Haya, while it was in the neighboring tribes. In the middle 1990s, a husband

and wife team, John and Pat Caldwell, mapped the progress of the AIDS epidemic in Africa. In elegant color maps, published in the Scientific American, they confirmed the work of Reining showing that the regions of Africa with the highest prevalence of HIV/AIDS coincided with the areas where the greatest numbers of males were uncircumcised. Other anthropologists who have been active in AIDS research include Drs. Daniel Halperin and Robert Bailey. Dr Halperin, in an article in Lancet entitled "Ten Years and Counting," questioned the lack of international action after 10 years of convincing evidence from multiple sources that circumcision protects against HIV infection.

And it is not in Africa alone that the link between HIV and male circumcision has been shown. There is a growing epidemic in Asia as well. A United Nations study (UNAIDS) looked at the varying prevalence of HIV in different regions of South and Southeast Asia and found similar results as in Africa. The regions where circumcision was practiced had markedly lower HIV rates than those where the men were uncircumcised.

Scientific documentation began in Kenya in 1988 when British researchers, working at a clinic for infectious diseases, found that men who were uncircumcised were almost 3 times more likely to acquire HIV as were circumcised men. These findings, published in the New England Journal of Medicine, lead them to conclude that "the intact foreskin may operate to increase the susceptibility to HIV." In 1989, another research group also working in Nairobi, Kenya, where 80% of the female prostitutes were infected with HIV, tested HIV-negative men 40 weeks after they'd had unprotected sex with these prostitutes. They showed that two factors increased the risk of HIV infection in the exposed men—either a sore on the penis due to a previously contracted infection (e.g., syphilis, chancroid, and herpes) or the presence of a foreskin.

Uncircumcised men had about 10 times the risk of becoming HIV positive as did circumcised men, and an uncircumcised man with a penile sore had 4 times the risk of a circumcised man with a similar lesion. The two risk factors were additive. A circumcised man with no penile sore had a 2.5% chance of becoming HIV positive, while an uncircumcised man with a penile sore had a 52% chance of acquiring HIV. Evidence from over 40 separate published studies has since confirmed these findings. A study in Rakai, Uganda added more proof of a link between circumcision and HIV. HIV-negative male partners of HIV- positive women were observed to see if they became HIV positive. There were 187 couples who were followed and tested. Of the 137 pairs in which the man was uncircumcised 40 of these men became infected with the HIV virus, while none of the 50 circumcised men became HIV positive. In India, a similarly impressive project showed that over a 7 year period in a clinic for sexually transmitted disease only 2 of 191 circumcised men (1.1%) became HIV-positive, while among the uncircumcised men the rate of HIV infection was almost 8 times higher. A number of researchers have recommended adult circumcision for all African men to halt the raging AIDS epidemic on that continent. A major carrier of HIV in Africa is the long distance truck driver who contracts the disease from prostitutes in big cities, then brings it back to his wife in the village, who in turn transmits it to the fetus and newborn. In the U.S., AIDS is still mainly a disease of gay men and intravenous drug abusers, although it is seen in heterosexual women as well as in children. The circumcision factor was found in 500 gay men in Seattle; those with foreskins had almost twice the risk of getting HIV infection as did their circumcised brethren.

There is a biologic explanation for the danger of the foreskin in acquiring HIV, just as is the case with urinary tract acquisition. But the methods of infection vary between the two diseases. As we have stated, UTIs are caused by specific bacteria with tentacles (uropathic organisms) which stick to the inner mucous membrane of the foreskin and ascend to the kidney to cause infection. In the case of HIV there is a different mechanism. Within the foreskin are large numbers of special HIV-specific target cells called CD4 T-lymphocytes and Langerhans cells, which are designed to trap and destroy invading germs. These target cells are effective in this search-and- destroy mission with most infecting organisms, but not with HIV. HIV is targeted and trapped very efficiently as with other invading germs, but there is a critical difference. The protective foreskin T-lymphocytes and Langerhans cells are unable to destroy the virus, which then enters the body. Convincing research studies, particularly by Dr. Roger Short at the University of Melbourne in Australia, have vividly shown this binding and trapping system by specialized cells present in large numbers in the foreskin, but not in the head of the penis (glans). There are added biologic mechanisms favoring circumcised men. The glans is covered by cells, which contain keratin, a protein that presents a barrier to viral entry. There is no such protective barrier in the foreskin. In addition, the delicate foreskin is more subject to tearing and abrasions than is the circumcised penis, and allows direct entry of the virus into the blood. Currently renowned investigators, leading health officials, and national and international organizations all accept the role of circumcision in HIV prevention. Dr Anthony Fauci, head of the HIV Research Division of the National Institutes of Health (NIH), stated that "the link between male circumcision and lower HIV infection rates is now absolute fact." The U.S. Agency for International Development (USAID) referred to "an incredible preponderance of evidence" of the protective effect of newborn circumcision. A United Nations study (UNAIDS) found from a two- to tenfold increase in HIV infection in regions of Asia and Africa where circumcision is not practiced compared to areas where it is.

In view of this overwhelming evidence, why is more not being done to implement large-scale circumcision in Africa? The answers are complex but there should be no excuse for inaction in the face of the HIV/AIDS disaster. HIV currently infects 46 million people in the world and over 20 million men, women and children have already died. There are 5 million new HIV cases and 3 million deaths annually. It is difficult to explain the reluctance by international health organizations to promote an intervention that leaves circumcised men 2-7 times less likely to acquire HIV than uncircumcised men. Is it excessive optimism that a vaccine or medical cure will be developed against this elusive and ever-changing virus? Is it an elitist attitude by wealthy, scientifically advanced countries unwilling to devote significant resources towards a disease that mainly affects poor, underdeveloped regions of the world? Is it a refusal to believe that a procedure used as a cultural/religious ritual can have valuable medical benefits? Is it the effectiveness of anti-circumcision activists? Is it cultural /religious bias? Probably a bit of all of the above. Regardless of the reasons, the sheer magnitude of the epidemic and unrelenting spread of HIV/AIDS warrant using circumcision as a weapon which has the potential to prevent millions of deaths. In 2000 Dr Malcolm Potts, a professor at the University of California in Berkeley, after reviewing the data of multiple studies, calculated that had all exposed men been circumcised there would have been 8 million fewer cases of HIV infection in the world—6 million in Africa and 2 million in Asia. More recently, Edward Green, a researcher of HIV at Harvard, estimated that if all males in Africa were circumcised the rate of HIV could be reduced from 20% to under 5%. Millions of lives would be saved.

It is understandable why circumcision was initially not considered as an intervention. In 1982 in the early years of the epidemic it was soon realized that having a foreskin was a risk factor in acquiring HIV infection. But the search was for complete protection and/or curative drugs. Things looked encouraging. The virus was isolated, a test developed, and it was expected that there would be a vaccine within 2 years. With other viral diseases, such as polio and measles, viral isolation usually meant a vaccine in the near future. Not so with HIV. There was not much trouble developing a vaccine against a predominant strain of HIV virus. The problem is that the virus was and is always one step ahead of the vaccine. Just when you think you have it, the virus mutates or "morphs" into another form, rendering the vaccine worthless or even risky. After years of trying, the vaccine seekers still don't have the answer. The drug path has been more successful, but the final solution is not at hand. The remarkable early success of AZT gave a new lease on life to AIDS sufferers waiting to die. But it soon became apparent that the virus was not going to stand still for AZT. As with the vaccines, drug-resistant mutants appeared, requiring the development of multiple anti-retroviral agents, so that today's AIDS victims are faced with a bewildering array of pills and treatment schedules. And the costs are high – probably too expensive for underdeveloped countries even with cheaper generics. Also, prevention is preferable to treatment and circumcision greatly improves the odds of not getting HIV in the first place. Almost 2 decades have been wasted looking for the ideal vaccine and drug treatment as the epidemic continues and millions die. Had mass circumcision programs, including newborns, been instituted in the early 1980s along with the search for vaccines and drugs millions of lives could have been saved. Also there would be a large population of young African men under the age of 20 who would now be less likely to acquire HIV on exposure.

Although there has been reluctance on the part of local and international organizations to encourage universal circumcision to help prevent the spread of HIV in Africa, there has been a very high rate of acceptability of circumcision among the Africans themselves. As was the case in the twin Zambian villages, the public seems to be ahead of the "experts" and official policy. In a series of surveys in Botswana and South Africa, areas of high HIV prevalence between 60-70% of uncircumcised men stated that they would want to be circumcised if the procedure could be done professionally and without cost.

In 2001 the potential for circumcision in fighting HIV was recognized in an article in the Botswana Guardian: "If in the year 1985, all Botswana men and boys had been circumcised, HIV/AIDS might never have reached pandemic proportions in this country. There can be no doubt that novel approaches are sorely needed to bring the AIDS pandemic to a close. The time has come in this country for public discussion about making circumcision widely available in clinics on a voluntary basis and strongly recommended for all boys under age 15." Klaits and Mogwe, *Botswana Guardian,* Jan. 2001.

Admittedly, a mass circumcision program in Africa presents major hurdles. There are not enough trained professionals to do the job. But the procedure is not difficult, and non-professionals could be trained to do circumcisions effectively and safely. The costs could be offset by savings on anti-retroviral drugs and other medical needs through prevention of HIV infection. There are some promising signs on the horizon. It is very encouraging that most uncircumcised young African men would be willing to undergo circumcision, even against their tribal tradition. USAID is now supporting the investigation of male circumcision as a tool in the fight against HIV/AIDS. We overlooked the value of circumcision in this battle in the past, with disastrous results. Let us not make this mistake again. Would there be such a cavalier attitude if the AIDS epidemic was occurring in the wealthier more advanced countries? The developed nations and international health organizations, such as the World Health Organization and the United Nations, should be in the forefront in promoting widespread circumcision to help control the HIV/AIDS epidemic. I don't think that the compelling evidence on the value of circumcision in HIV prevention would be ignored if the foreskin/HIV relationship was discovered in the twin cities of Minneapolis and St. Paul or Buda and Pest rather than in Lozi and Luvale in Zambia.

6

Other Sexually Transmitted Diseases (STDs)

A known scourge for centuries, syphilis was known as the "White Plague" in the middle ages to distinguish it from the "Black (Bubonic) Plague." It was the AIDS of its day. Millions died from it, and it invaded every tissue of the body, from the bones to the brain, leading to crippling, paralysis and mental deterioration, and finally to death. It attacked men, women and newborn babies. The British and Italians called it "the French Disease" (Francophobia is not a new phenomenon). As a medical student and pediatric intern in New York City in the late 1940s I recall vividly seeing cases of infants born with congenital syphilis, a common disease on the eve of the discovery of penicillin. Every medical student of that era had seen many cases of congenital syphilis. In these desperately ill newborns, we learned to quickly make the diagnosis by the typical skin rashes, the mucous membrane secretions, involvement of many organs, and the moth-eaten look of the bones on X-Ray. These are findings that young pediatricians of today likely have never seen, and, happily, never will in a lifetime of practice. By examining secretions and body fluids we could quickly prove that syphilis was present simply by seeing hordes of the wiggling, corkscrew-shaped spirochetes through a microscope. It was fortunate that by the time I was in my second year of pediatric specialty training we had penicillin and that spelled the virtual end of the scourge of syphilis. But routine syphilis testing is an important part of preventive medical care—think of all pregnant women being tested, and the premarital requirement. We have to remain vigilant against the mini-outbreaks of syphilis that we still see periodically, so that early treatment will prevent congenital syphilis.

In comparing syphilis and HIV, there is good news and bad news. They both are epidemic STD's that engender terror in large populations. They both affect men, women and children, and pregnant women can pass it on to the infant. That could be considered to be the good news, since we have essentially beaten syphilis, and the fear is largely gone. The bad news is that HIV/AIDS is tougher to fight. Syphilis, in its infectious stages, can be diagnosed by seeing the spirochetes under a microscope. HIV is invisible and elusive. The syphilis spirochete is not very smart or adaptable. It has been over 50 years since penicillin came along and it still kills the germ, which has not learned to develop resistance or mutate. HIV continually mutates and changes itself. For over 20 years it has frustrated attempts to develop a magic bullet to kill it once and for all, or to develop an effective vaccine. By using as models the complete cure of syphilis by penicillin, and the success in developing vaccines against other viral diseases, investigators of HIV/AIDS have devoted all their efforts to anti-HIV drugs and vaccines. The preventive effect of circumcision has been ignored in the hope of getting a complete cure, thus losing the opportunity to save millions of lives at the same time as the drive to cure the disease continues.

As with HIV, the foreskin is an important portal of entry for syphilis. This is not recent news. It has been known for centuries that Jews and other circumcised groups are less likely to get syphilis when exposed. Remarkably, the mechanism by which the foreskin acts as a risk factor for getting syphilis was described in the 1500's, during the European syphilis epidemic. Gabriello Fallopia, an Italian anatomist stated that: "Men with a long foreskin and a covered glans can be contaminated (by syphilis) more easily because they are more tender and there receive the virus (sic) more easily." This observation has been repeatedly confirmed over the centuries. Dr R.Wilson, reviewing experience with STDs in the Canadian Army after World War II, wrote: "tears and abrasions of the foreskin are commonly seen on sick parade. Small abrasions of the delicate coronal membrane occur during brothel intercourse. Both provide a portal of entry for the spirochete." Almost identical words to those of Fallopia 500 years earlier. In 1988, in a large controlled study at an STD clinic in Seattle, it was found that the odds of uncircumcised men getting syphilis on exposure were 4 times as great as in circumcised men. In a wide-ranging analysis of "conventional" STDs, Dr. Stephen Moses found that in 11 separate research projects on syphilis circumcision helped prevent the disease in exposed men in all of the studies. Circumcision also aided in the prevention of chancroid, an STD with a sore on the penis very similar to the chancre of syphilis. During the Korean War it was found that 90% of the cases of chancroid in U.S. soldiers occurred in uncircumcised men, who made up only 33% of the men.

Not long ago I was reminded of the ease with which the delicate foreskin is torn. A concerned mother of a 4-year-old boy wondered why her son was complaining of penile discomfort. Exam showed a very tender foreskin, not fully retractable, with a number of breaks in the skin surface, which could easily allow entry of an aggressive microbe. Simple lubrication was all that was necessary at this time. A decade or two later, when this boy becomes sexually active, his tight, delicate, easily torn foreskin will place him at greater risk of getting syphilis, chancroid, and human papilloma virus

(HPV) and genital herpes, as well as HIV, all of which are STDs which can enter through a damaged foreskin. The uncovered penis with its tougher surface, covered with keratinized cells, is much less easily damaged and blocks entry of these STDs. In the case of gonorrhea the foreskin promotes entry of the bacteria by another means. The area between the foreskin and the glans provides a warm moist area in which infecting organisms can easily grow. The gonorrhea bacteria thrive under the foreskin and enter the urethral opening at the end of the penis where they set up house and multiply, leading to the characteristic thick yellow discharge. If left untreated this infection becomes chronic, leading to scarring and narrowing of the urethral tube ("stricture"). This blocking stricture causes difficult, painful urination, and may have to be treated by stretching with metal tubes ("sounds"), a very unpleasant procedure, but one that was often necessary in the pre-antibiotic days. Hopefully, gonorrhea doesn't progress to this stage nowadays, but it can lead to serious consequences when passed on to female sexual partners. In women, gonorrhea causes an internal infection, pelvic inflammatory disease (PID), which involves inflammation and possible permanent blockage of the fallopian tubes, often causing sterility.

The thought of males with sore, scraped foreskins brings me back five decades to my time as a young naval flight surgeon on aircraft carriers during the Korean conflict. One of my medical duties when the ship dropped anchor in a foreign port was to go ashore and set up an area to try to head off STDs, a "pro station." Two visits to the pro station were required of all sailors, one "prior to," on coming ashore and one "just after" sexual exposure, before returning to the ship. The preliminary visit was straightforward; abstinence was advised, and condoms and hygiene instructions were issued, usually to be ignored. The return contact prior to reboarding ship was more complex, often being conducted amidst varying shades of sobriety and hostility. This phallic exit poll consisted of a genital exam known as a "short arm inspection" in Navy parlance. Inspection was followed by the infusion of an antiseptic solution into the urethra, sort of a penile enema. I looked at many exit poll penises, most of which were circumcised, and it was obvious that the uncircumcised ones were worse for wear, often scratched and weeping like the nose of the family dog who has gone a few rounds with the neighborhood cat. On the other hand the circumcised penis might look either shiny or ruddy like W.C. Field's nose or a bit shriveled like a Santa Clara prune, but the surface was intact, acting as a barrier to invading infections. There was also no warm moist area in which germs could grow.

Thus, as is the case with HIV, the proof is overwhelming and beyond a reasonable doubt that the presence of a foreskin increases the risk of acquiring syphilis and chancroid. But what about the other STDs, including gonorrhea, the human papilloma virus (HPV), genital herpes and nongonorrheal urethritis (a common disease usually caused by Chlamydia)? Is the uncircumcised man more likely to get these STDs? Here, depending upon the condition, the evidence varies from very strong for HPV, to so-so for genital herpes and gonorrhea, to absent in the case of Chlamydia infection.

The most significant of these infecting agents is HPV, a virus that has been shown to be "oncogenic," meaning that its action on cells can lead to cancer. HPV has been implicated in both cervical cancer and penile cancer, having been repeatedly isolated from both of these lethal tumors. In a recent important multinational analysis of cervical cancer, reported in the *New England Journal of Medicine*, uncircumcised men were found to be 3 times as likely to be carrying HPV as circumcised men, and cervical cancer was more commonly seen in female partners of uncircumcised men. Because it is so common, HPV may be the most important STD in the U.S. today, but its importance is not in its effect on the man who is carrying it beneath his foreskin. Although chronic HPV infection may be the causative factor for penile cancer, cervical cancer is about 10 times more common, so the male carrier of HPV is more of a danger to his female sexual partner(s) than he is to himself.

With gonorrhea, it's not the delicate foreskin that allows the infection to progress, but rather the warm, moist environment under the foreskin which favors bacterial growth and allows the organisms to multiply and contaminate the urethral opening and mucosa. Of the 7 research studies on gonorrhea analyzed by Dr. Moses, circumcision was protective in 5, and seemed to have no effect in 2. The warmth and moisture under the foreskin doesn't seem to be as favorable for Chlamydia, the main cause of non-gonorrheal urethritis since there is no evidence of a favorable effect of circumcision on this STD. Presence of the foreskin in genital herpes in 214 men in White Chapel Clinic in London was compared with 410 controls from the same clinic, and circumcision was found to have a significant protective effect.

So in looking at STDs, we now know from multiple studies that, in addition to HIV, circumcision definitely protects against syphilis and chancroid. There is strong evidence that it helps prevent genital herpes and HPV infection, but there is no beneficial action against non-gonorrheal urethritis. The general conclusion is that the foreskin puts a man at high risk for certain STDs, particularly the most serious ones—HIV, syphilis and HPV.

7

Cancer of the Penis

When Diego Rivera, the great Mexican muralist, died of cancer of the penis in 1957, it was a double tragedy. Not only had he suffered from a lethal disease, but as a man of great libido, the loss of sexual prowess had been devastating. He refused the usual treatment—partial penile amputation. Instead, the dedicated Communist went to Moscow for radiation therapy, which resulted in considerable discomfort and tissue damage, but failed to arrest the progress of his malignancy. His faith in the Soviet system might have been shaken by this experience. He suffered a painful death with spread of the cancer throughout his body.

Penile cancer is almost exclusively a disease of uncircumcised men. Rivera was uncircumcised, since circumcision is not practiced in Latin America and in much of the rest of the world outside the United States, except among Muslims and Jews. Newborn circumcision offers almost complete protection against cancer of the penis. Of the 50,000 cases of penile cancer in the U.S. over the past half-century, only 10 were reported in circumcised men. That's about 1000 cases yearly in uncircumcised men and only 1 reported case every 5 years in circumcised men, despite the fact that most U.S. men are circumcised. Overwhelming evidence. No need for statistics here. The effect of penile cancer on the health of American men cannot be compared to breast cancer in women, since it is many times less common. But while a cure for breast cancer seems far in the future, given the complexities of genes, environment, early diagnosis, and multiple treatment, cancer of the penis could be just about completely eliminated in one fell swoop by a quick, simple, preventive procedure—universal newborn circumcision.

It has been known for over a century that penile cancer is a disease of uncircumcised men, and that newborn circumcision essentially eliminates the chance of getting this devastating cancer. In a 1932 survey of all United States hospitals 1103 cases of cancer of the penis were identified. None of the men were circumcised. Three years later, in 1935, at the cancer hospital in New York City which is now Sloan Kettering Institute a renowned urologist, Dr. A. J. Dean, reported 120 cases of penile cancer. Again, they were all in uncircumcised men. Dean, sensing the potential for the elimination of penile cancer stated; "The prophylactic treatment of cancer of the penis consists in circumcising all male infants a few days after birth." Since then there have been at least 6 major studies from all over the U.S., each with between 78 and 156 men with penile cancer, encompassing over 600 cases, all in uncircumcised men. In 1973, almost 40 years after Dean's work, Dagher, who reported the largest of these penile cancer series, echoed the continued frustration of urologists; "Despite overwhelming evidence from urologic surgeons that neoplasm of the penis is a lethal disease that can be prevented by removal of the foreskin, some physicians continue to argue against routine neonatal circumcision in a highly emotional and aggressive fashion."

Although every study on the subject of penile cancer has found that circumcision protects against this lethal malignancy, a single study from Washington state, claimed that the protection was not as great as thought, with uncircumcised men only 3 times more likely to get the disease. This study had serious methodological flaws the most significant of which was that the malignant disease, invasive penile cancer (IPC), was lumped together with a benign disorder, carcinoma in situ (CIS). We looked into this issue among 213 men (91 with IPC and 122 with CIS), diagnosed with these disorders over a 43 year period (1954-1997) in Kaiser Permanente, a large California Health Maintenance Organization (HMO). Our report, published in 2000, found that there was indeed a threefold risk of uncircumcised men getting the benign form of the disease (CIS), but the uncircumcised men were more than 20 times as likely to get the malignant form (IPC). Not only that, but the rare malignant cases in circumcised men were milder and occurred in older men. Of the 89 invasive cancer cases only 2 were in circumcised men. These men were ages 79 and 84 years when the diagnosis was made (average age of uncircumcised IPC cases was 64), they had early disease treated with simple excision rather than with penectomy, and they were alive and well 8 and 3 years after surgery. It is not valid to lump together the benign and malignant forms of the disease when analyzing the protective effect of circumcision. Newborn circumcision helps prevent the benign, precancerous form of penile cancer, but it virtually eliminates the malignant disease.

Good genital hygiene helps prevent cancer of the penis, but it is an aid to circumcision, not a substitute. In looking at the world, the lowest rates of penile cancer are in countries and regions with good genital hygiene in addition to circumcision. The highest rates are in areas where there is poor genital hygiene and the men are uncircumcised, with in-between values in countries with one or the other. The International Agency for Research on Cancer (IARC) studied the incidence of penile cancer (cases per 100,000 males) in 5 continents. The lowest incidence, with a value of 0.1, was in Israel, a country with a high standard of hygiene in which essentially all the males are circumcised in the newborn period.

The highest rates of cancer were in Paraguay (4.2) and parts of Rhodesia (8.6), incidences 42 and 86 times greater than in Israel. Western European countries, with good hygiene but no circumcision had intermediate values (1.0 and 0.9 in Denmark and Germany), values about 10 times as high as Israel. The situation is more complex in the U.S., where the incidence value (1.0), is a mixture of low incidence in circumcised men and high incidence in uncircumcised men. This is illustrated by the differences between Puerto Ricans and Filipinos living in the U.S. Both groups are at about the same socio-economic level, but the Filipinos have their sons circumcised while the Puerto Ricans do not. The incidence of penile cancer in the U.S. Filipinos (0.1) is 30 times less than in the U.S. Puerto Ricans (3.0). So don't believe it when you hear that you don't need circumcision to prevent penile cancer as long as there is good genital hygiene. It's best if you have both, but circumcision is number one in importance as measured by incidence rates.

There is strong evidence that penile cancer, like cervical cancer, is an infectious, sexually transmitted disease (Chapters 6,8). The same virus, the human papilloma virus (HPV) is involved in both penile and cervical cancer. And not just HPV, but specific subtypes of HPV, particularly HPV type 16, and, to a lesser extent, type 18. HPV can cause genital warts, but it is usually present with no outward evidence. HPV is said to be the most common of all STDs, being carried on the penis of about 6% of men. In an important recent study of cervical cancer, which will be described more fully in the Chapter on Cervical Cancer (Chapter 8), it was found that uncircumcised men are 3 times more likely to have HPV on the penis than are circumcised men. In a South American study HPV16 was found in 43% of penile cancers, and HPV18 in an additional 9%, so that HPV was isolated in over half of penile cancer tissue. Populations with high rates

of penile cancer have high rates of cervical cancer and the men
are uncircumcised. In India, where there are Muslims, who circumcise, and Hindus, who do not, the results in almost 5000
cervical cancer cases and 300 men with penile cancer showed
that none of the penile cancer cases were in Muslims, and the
incidence of cervical cancer was 2.5 times as great in the Hindu
women compared to Muslim women. Since cervical cancer is
much more common in the world than is penile cancer, it seems
likely that an uncircumcised man, as a source of HPV, presents
more of a threat of causing cervical cancer to his female partner
than he does of getting penile cancer himself. A circumcised
man on the other hand not only has almost no risk of getting
penile cancer, but he is less likely to be harboring the papilloma
virus and passing it on to a female sexual partner where it can
lead to cervical cancer. Male circumcision protects against genital cancer in both sexes.

In view of the benefit of circumcision in preventing genital
cancer it would seem logical for governments and medical
professional organizations to encourage the procedure, but
this is not the case. The American Academy of Pediatrics,
in the latest pronouncement in 1999 does not recommend
routine newborn circumcision. The National Health Service
in England does not pay for newborn circumcision, leading
to a rapid decline in rate of circumcision in that country over
the past 50 years since the program was instituted. Canada
and Australia have followed suit. Has that had an effect on
the incidence of penile cancer in these countries? This is a
difficult question to answer, because it takes 40-60 years for
penile cancer to develop. But in 1990 an Australian study
looked at this issue in 102 cases seen from 1953-1984, and
found that the incidence of penile cancer was twice as great
in the last decade after circumcision was discontinued as it
was after the first decade, concluding that infant circumcision is the best policy to prevent penile cancer.

8

Cancer of the Cervix in Female Partners

When Eva Peron, wife of the dictator Juan Peron, died of cervical cancer at age 32, Argentina cried for her, particularly the poor. The powerful Evita presented herself as a champion of the common people against the upper classes. Born in poverty, a child of the streets, she clawed her way to the top, some say on her back, by liaisons with influential men, mainly in the military. Although her ascent to national leadership and international fame was rare and remarkable for a woman of her background, her disease was not. She had a lifestyle typical for a woman who will develop cancer of the cervix early in life. The usual victim begins sexual activity at a young age, often in the pre-teens and has had multiple sexual partners. This lethal cancer is common in prostitutes and almost unheard of in nuns. Early sexual activity subjects a vulnerable cervix to injury from trauma, and multiple sexual partners increase the risk of acquiring human papilloma virus (HPV) infection. HPV has been implicated as the causative agent of cervical cancer. And HPV is more commonly carried by uncircumcised men.

It is not possible to talk about cervical cancer without bringing in penile cancer. In assessing risk factors for cervical cancer in Denmark in 1991, Dr. S. K. Kael characterized a "high risk male partner" as one who is uncircumcised, doesn't use condoms, and has a history of genital warts and multiple sexual partners. In other words one who is carrying the human papilloma virus (HPV) on his penis. Further we now know the viruses most commonly involved are HPV types 16 or 18. From the standpoint of developing genital cancer, the male HPV carrier is more of a risk to women partners than he is to himself. In the large series of genital cancers from Madras, India, there were almost 5000 cervical cancer cases and only 300 cases of penile cancer, a ratio of 16 to 1. Cervical cancer made up 35% of all female cancers, while penile cancer represented only 2.7% of male cancers. All of the 300 men with penile cancer were Hindus or Christians, who are uncircumcised—none were Muslims, who practice circumcision. Cervical cancer was 2.5 times as common in Hindu women and 1.9 times as common in Christian women as it was in the Muslim women. The authors concluded that circumcision is important in reducing the risk of both penile and cervical cancer. To speculate on these data, one could conclude that an uncircumcised man, through carriage of HPV, is 16 times more likely to cause cervical cancer in a female partner than he is to get penile cancer himself. Failure to recommend circumcision on the basis of the fact that penile cancer is such a rare disease ignores the evidence of female transmission, not to mention the many other disorders prevented by newborn circumcision. Cervical cancer is the second most common cancer in women. There are about 500,000 cervical cancer cases in the world every year, with nearly a quarter of a million deaths. In the United States there are 13,000 cases and 4100 deaths annually, a figure 10 to 20 times greater than penile cancer.

The relationship between lack of circumcision, penile cancer, and cervical cancer has been known for over 100 years through population studies. Ethnic and religious groups that circumcise have less genital cancer than those who do not.

Jews and Muslims have low rates and Hindus have high rates of both penile and cervical cancer. In 1936, in the Fiji Islands, where some groups circumcise and some do not, it was found that those islanders who do not practice religious circumcision have an incidence of genital cancer 8 times as great as those who do.

There has been evidence, now irrefutable, for about 50 years that cervical and penile cancers are sexually transmitted diseases. Cervical cancer was induced in mice in 1958 by the repeated application of human smegma to the cervix and vagina. It was felt that this tumor-producing effect of smegma was mediated through sex-borne infection and chronic inflammation. No viral isolation techniques were available at the time, but there was reference to the "virus theory of human cancer." By the 1970s it was realized that the papilloma viruses could produce tumors in various hosts. Special surface cells ("stratified squamous epithelium") were particularly vulnerable, including those on the penis, cervix and vaginal wall. The 1980s represented the era of the specific isolation and characterization of the subtypes of human papilloma virus (HPV).In an important publication in 1986 entitled "Human papilloma virus and cancer" D.J. McCance, a researcher at Guy's Hospital in London, clearly described convincing evidence gathered by himself and others that closely linked specific types of HPV, particularly HPV 16 and HPV 18, to both penile and cervical cancer. In Brazil, HPV 16 was isolated from 50% of penile cancers. At about the same time, a report from Paris, where newborn circumcision is not performed, found a high incidence of abnormal cells on the penises of male sex partners of women with precancerous lesions of the cervix. HPV 16 was isolated from most of these lesions in both sexes, and often the same HPV type was found on the penis and cervix of sexual partners. Certain genital warts ("flat warts") are caused by "high risk" HPV types, mainly HPV 16 and 18 and are precursors of cancer, while other warts (condyloma accuminata) are usually caused by HPV types 6 and 11 and are considered benign.

During the 1990s the evidence continued to accumulate showing that cancer of the cervix and penis were sexually transmitted. Methods for isolating and typing HPV improved, allowing for more clinical observations. It was pointed out that cervical cancer may be the first human malignancy for which we have isolated a single, necessary causative factor, the human papilloma virus. HPV 16 was found responsible for about 50% of cervical cancers, and four types (HPV 16, 18, 31 and 45) accounted for 80%, with the rest divided among the more than 30 HPV types.

In 2002, two exciting landmark studies on cervical cancer were published in the *New England Journal of Medicine,* and both were thought to be worthy of editorial comment. The first came from the Cancer Institute in Barcelona, Spain and was an analysis of data pooled from 7 separate well-performed (case-control) studies from 5 countries reported by the International Agency for Research on Cancer over a 15 year period. The investigators, Castellsague and his colleagues, analyzed the relationship between male circumcision, penile HPV infection and cervical cancer in female partners. They found that penile HPV was present in 166 of the 847 uncircumcised men (19.6%), but in only 16 of the 292 circumcised men (5.5%). Uncircumcised men were 3 times as likely to be carrying the causative agent of cervical cancer as were circumcised men. In the case of men with multiple sexual partners, there was a twofold reduced risk of cervical cancer in the current female partner if the man was circumcised, a significant cancer protection compared to uncircumcised men. This convincing study was followed within a few months by an analysis of the effectiveness of a vaccine against HPV 16 in preventing cervical cancer. In a controlled study involving almost 2400 young women in a number of medical centers in the U.S., Koutsky and collaborators found that the HPV 16 vaccine reduced the incidence not only of HPV 16 infection but also of precancerous HPV-related cervical abnormalities (intraepithelial neoplasia). The editorial commenting on this important work was entitled "The Beginning of the End for Cervical Cancer?" Let us be optimistic and hope that the question mark will disappear, but we must be cautious before we start celebrating the success of this vaccine prematurely, as the editorial writer pointed out. This was a preliminary study, and hopes for an effective vaccine have been dashed before—think of HIV. Hopefully HPV 16 will not mutate and stay ahead of the vaccine. Also, it must be remembered that there are other types of HPV that can cause cervical cancer, although HPV 16 is the most important. Then there is the question of whom to target for vaccination, young women before they become sexually active, or everyone, male and female, in order to reduce the carrier state in men. It will take at least 10 years to notice a reduction in cervical cancer, so the effectiveness will not be immediately apparent. If things work out, perhaps a vaccine could be made to include HPV 18, as well as HPV 6 and 11 to prevent genital warts. The potential is great, and we can be optimistic though not overly enthusiastic, at least not so far.

Demographic changes in the U.S. add to the importance of the circumcision factor in preventing cervical cancer. In 2000 there were about 35 million Hispanics in this country, comprising 12.5% of the total population, up from 9% in 1990. Hispanics are the fastest growing minority group in the U.S. There is a high rate of cervical cancer in Hispanic women, as illustrated by Eva Peron, and Hispanics generally do not have their boys circumcised. This is particularly apparent in California, where the total newborn circumcision rate has fallen in half over the past 20 years, from a value of 70% to the current level of less than 40%, compared to a circumcision rate of 80% in the Midwestern states. The falling California circumcision rate is not due to success of the anti-circumcision groups, which are so active in the state (the non-Hispanic circumcision rate is still about 70%), but simply reflects the fact that currently Hispanic infants comprise over 50% of the more than 500,000 infants born each year in California. If none of the Hispanic boys are circumcised, the circumcision rate for the state would be less than 50% even if 100% of non-Hispanic infant boys were circumcised. And the cervical cancer rate in Hispanic women is high. Women in Mexico, Central and South America have approximately triple the mortality rate from cervical cancer as do women in the U.S. Within the U.S., in the period from 1992-1999 the incidence for invasive cervical cancer in Hispanic women was about twice that of non-Hispanic women (16.9 vs. 8.9 per100, 000 women). This is bothersome. As the population of Hispanics in the U.S. continues to rise we can expect to see more cervical cancer. That is, unless Hispanic males choose circumcision. There is some encouragement along this line. Although very few Hispanic newborn boys are circumcised in the areas closest to the Mexican border, there seems to be more acceptance as the migration proceeds to the North. Recently it was found that 29% of Hispanic males born at San Francisco General Hospital were circumcised. As with other immigrant groups, there is pressure for increased conformity to U.S. standards as time passes. In the meantime there should be increased efforts to make sure that Hispanic women are screened frequently for cervical cancer with pap smears.

As with HIV, the final solution to cervical cancer will be the elimination of the causative virus, either through effective anti-viral medication, or preferably through vaccination. But in the meantime we know that circumcision of male sexual partners reduces the risk of cervical cancer twofold in developed countries and up to eightfold in underdeveloped countries. An intact foreskin increases the chances of both penile and cervical cancer. Worldwide universal circumcision could prevent hundreds of thousands of deaths annually from cervical cancer.

9

Sex and Sensitivity

Never mind about health benefits and disease prevention. Never mind about improved cleanliness. The big question is what does the foreskin do for SEX?

Does having a foreskin give a man an advantage or a disadvantage in the sexual arena? And how do women feel about it? We hear from men who have been circumcised at birth and complain that they are missing out by not having a foreskin. But how would they know? The men who should have the answers are those who have had it both ways – they have had sex with foreskins and then been circumcised as adults. Well let's hear a couple of true life stories:

Case 1: "I was 23 when I decided to get circumcised. Although my foreskin moved back and forth, I still had an odor from the smegma sometime. Having sex with a foreskin was the worst thing that could have happened. After the circumcision what more can I say but I love it. It is the best thing that I could have done for myself. Sex and masturbation is (sic) absolutely wonderful. I love being a clean cut circumcised man. I feel so much more confident in myself and I am no longer embarrassed in any way about my manhood." Internet correspondence, 2003.

Case 2: "I am 27 years old and was circumcised 2 years ago for no medical reason. I wished to look like everyone else. I never had an infection or a problem of any kind. Since the operation my glans is far less sensitive. I have a problem with premature ejaculation which I never had. Sex is far less pleasurable, and masturbation a horror." Personal correspondence, 1989.

There you have it. Sex with a foreskin is better. Sex with a foreskin is worse. Masturbation after circumcision becomes "absolutely wonderful" or it becomes a "horror." Case 2 states that after circumcision his glans was less sensitive, which makes some sense, but why would he be having premature ejaculation, which is attributed to more penile sensitivity? But in this field logic doesn't always win.

Between 1987 and 1989, as Chairman of the American Academy of Pediatrics (AAP) Task Force on Circumcision, I received carloads of correspondence containing opinions and personal experiences relating the foreskin to sexual activity. In Chapter 11 I will share more of these anecdotes with you, but I can sum them up by saying you can find testimonials to support any viewpoint you favor. Like the examples above, some correspondents said that their sex life was rejuvenated after adult circumcision, while others blamed their parents for having them circumcised since it ruined their chances for later normal sexual activity. Anti–circumcision groups refer to circumcision as "male genital mutilation" and have blamed it for everything from impotence to emotional instability and major psychological disorders. On the basis of research data there is no evidence that the foreskin affects sexual function one way or the other in either gender. There is one exception, and that is in the case of oral sex, where female correspondents overwhelmingly prefer the circumcised penis for reasons having to do with genital hygiene.

We can look at large populations of either circumcised or uncircumcised men to try to find differences. For instance there are over 100 million circumcised males in the United States. Is there any evidence to indicate that U.S. men have less sexual pleasure than do say Russian or Swedish men? Or that Russian or Swedish women are better satisfied sexually than are U.S. women? Not that I could discover. As a matter of fact during World War II American GIs, most of whom were circumcised, did just fine with European women. There didn't seem to be a sense of loss on the part of these women that no foreskin was present. Many expressed their feelings by becoming war brides, with no evidence that they were missing something. There also doesn't seem to be any observed differences in sexual function in India between Muslims, who are circumcised, and Hindus, who are not. Both groups seem to do fine, well, sexually. But aren't there at least some studies out there? Fortunately there are, particularly in the past few years, and I will share them with you, as well as some opinions of correspondents that I have found interesting.

In 1988 a husband and wife team named Williamson assessed the preference of circumcision status for various sexual activities in women in middle America (Iowa City).Using 4 criteria, they asked these women whether they preferred the circumcised or uncircumcised penis for sexual intercourse, to cause arousal by looking, for giving manual stimulation and for performing oral sex. Some women had no preference, but 71% preferred the circumcised penis for sexual intercourse compared to 6% for the uncircumcised organ. For the other activities it was 76% circumcised vs. 4% uncircumcised for looking, and 75% vs. 5% for manual stimulation. The greatest preference for the circumcised man was in oral sex with 83% preferring the circumcised penis and only 2% favoring the uncircumcised one. Having gotten these impressive results in favor of circumcision, the Williamsons then went on to ask those preferring the circumcised penis why they did so. The answers were it stays cleaner (92%), it looks sexier (90%), it feels nicer (85%), and a fourth reason which was most surprising of all, and should be most disturbing to those favoring the preservation of the foreskin. Believe it or not, a clear majority of these women (77%) thought that the circumcised penis looked "more natural." It seems as if even Mother Nature is in the eye of the beholder.

A less formal survey was carried out in 1996 in the London Times by its medical editor, Dr. T. Stuttiford. The subjects were "experienced women" and prostitutes, those most qualified to know. It was found that 90% of these women preferred sex with circumcised men because it was more hygienic and pleasurable.

Two well known women writers, Rachel Swift and Anne Lamott have weighed in on the subject. In the opinion of Ms. Swift: "The male member is not a thing of beauty; it has a tendency to smell unless the floppy bit at the end is cut off." She felt that circumcision is a must for oral sex. As mentioned previously Lamott also commented on the appearance of the uncircumcised penis comparing it to rodents caught in a garden hose.

That's how women feel. What about men? In a survey of 1410 men, ages 18-59, Laumann found that circumcised men engage in more elaborate sexual practices and uncircumcised men are more likely to experience sexual dysfunction especially later in life. But you won't get acceptance of these findings by a large body of vocal male anti-circumcisionists who claim that their erectile dysfunction is due to the fact that their parents had them circumcised as newborns. They feel that the center of sexual pleasure resides in that small piece of skin which they lost in infancy. The head of the penis (glans) must be covered at all costs to ensure sexual competence. Some of these men have been so dedicated to the cause that they have undergone a prolonged surgical procedure and had skin grafted to the end of the penis to cover the glans, producing sort of a foreskin look-alike. Others have attempted to stretch the skin of their circumcised penis by attaching various devices to the shaft, including lead weights and rubber bands. In the well-reviewed German language film *Europa, Europa,* the protagonist was an Aryan-appearing adolescent Jewish boy attempting to maintain his identity as a model member of a Hitler Youth group. He was understandably fearful that if he was observed naked his circumcised penis would betray him. His attempts to stretch the skin on his penis were not very successful as I recall, but he used other creative means to survive. We can empathize with the motivation of this young man to create something looking like a foreskin, since it was a life or death matter, but I fail to see the logic in current day America where circumcised men are not sent to crematory ovens.

By far the commonest claim among circumcised anti-circumcision men is that they have erectile dysfunction, an inability to perform sexually, and the reason is because the essential organ for normal sexual function, the foreskin, was taken from them in infancy. It was beyond their control, and their civil rights were violated. Some express anger at their parents for having them "mutilated." This anger and resentment often result in many forms of activism. Currently there is a web site on the Internet in which a 34 year old man, claiming impotence which he attributes to newborn circumcision, is attempting to get before Congress a bill to ban male circumcision in this country. He calls it the "MGM bill"—nothing to do with a movie studio. MGM stands for Male Genital Mutilation. Given the strong preference of the American public in favor of newborn circumcision, I wouldn't bet on this bill, and I see no evidence of congressmen in an election year rushing to embrace a ban on a procedure favored by 75% of voters.

The intensity with which activists try to advance the anti-circumcision cause and the depth of their feelings was revealed to me in a disturbing way in 1996. I had published articles, and performed research studies on the medical effects of new-born circumcision, which showed substantial health bene-fits of the procedure. At the time I had been mentioned in the media frequently, and was often asked to speak before medical groups. It was well known that I was a proponent of newborn circumcision. A writer for the *Reader's Digest,* Edwin Kiester, was doing a piece for the magazine on the topic and asked to interview me. I was scheduled to give a lecture on newborn circumcision before a joint meeting of the Pediatrics and Obstetric departments of our hospital, and I invited him to attend. Since the medical conferences at our hospital are posted in a number of locations, the local anti-circumcision organizations must have gotten wind of it. On the day of my talk, about 10-15 members of the larg-est local anti-circumcision group (of which there are quite a few in the San Francisco Bay Area) formed a picket line around the hospital, carrying plaques condemning circumci-sion. About 50 physicians showed up at my lecture, many of whom I knew, but I noticed some unfamiliar faces in the audience. The conference was uneventful until I finished my presentation and the question period began. It became ap-parent that the unfamiliar faces in the hall were members of anti-circumcision groups, since a number rose to express opposition to circumcision. Finally, a very large man arose to testify that he had sexual dysfunction, and this was due to his newborn circumcision. He blamed his parents, but he felt that the main culprits were physicians who encouraged circumcision. He had started talking fairly calmly, but as he went on he became more and more agitated. He began to advance menacingly towards the lecture podium to my con-sternation and the concern of the *Reader's Digest* writer who was in the first row, close to me. Fortunately we had a quick-thinking moderator who immediately ended the conference, people started to stand up impeding the way to the podium and cooler heads among the man's compatriots were able to calm him down. The writer was duly impressed with the intensity of feelings about circumcision. The *Reader's Digest* article appeared in July 1996, but no reference was made to the unplanned grand finale. Fortunately, that was the only time I have felt threatened physically, although I have periodically been the recipient of verbal and written threats from anti-circumcision sources.

Well, how much credence should we give to the claims that circumcision spoils sex? Not much. To the claimants, they have erectile dysfunction and they are circumcised, so the two must be related. But what about the millions of U.S. males who are circumcised and are great sexual performers?

Masters and Johnson, in their 1965 best selling book *Human Sexual Response,* reported a study of 35 uncircumcised and 35 circumcised men tested for penile sensitivity using a variety of neurological measurements. They found no differences between the 2 groups. Recently even more compelling research data and objective reports have been published in medical journals. In 2002, 2 studies appeared in the main urologic journal, the Journal of Urology, both of which were performed on U.S. men and concluded that circumcision has no overall significant effect on sexual performance. We could quibble on a few minor issues. In one study 15 sexually active men were surveyed before circumcision and 12 weeks after the procedure. There was no difference in sex drive, erection, ejaculation or overall satisfaction. No effect here. In the other project, 128 men who had been circumcised as adults, at an average age of 42 years, were questioned. The results were more equivocal. There was thought to be some decrease in sensitivity and erectile function after circumcision. But, on the other hand sexual satisfaction was improved and there was no change in sexual activity. Less sensitivity and erectile function but better sexual satisfaction? Difficult to draw conclusions. In 2004 in Turkey, 42 men were circumcised, mainly for religious reasons (Muslims circumcise, but different sects do it at different ages), at an average age of 22 years. They were evaluated using a more formal test of sexual function, the BMSFI (Brief Male Sexual Function Inventory) as well as a measurement of ejaculatory latency time. These evaluations were done before circumcision and 12 weeks after. There was no significant difference in the BMSFI before and after circumcision. On the other hand, there was a significantly longer ejaculatory latency time after circumcision. These authors concluded that adult circumcision does not adversely affect sexual function. As a matter of fact the increased time to reach ejaculation could be considered to be an advantage. Longer sex is better sex.

So, on the basis of recent clinical research, as contrasted with anecdotal comments, there is no evidence that the foreskin has any significant effect on sexual function. If anything, sex seems to become more pleasurable and variable after circumcision. This should not surprise us. The idea that the center of sex is in the foreskin is a naïve, simplistic idea, embraced by lay opponents of circumcision with no knowledge of the complex nature of sexual function.

The sexual act results from a technical cascade of events involving multiple biologic systems, including those in the brain, spinal cord, and circulatory system, which are mediated by many hormonal and enzymatic factors. Sexual feelings all start with the processing of sexual stimulation, manual and psychological, by the brain, and are transmitted by nerve impulses and chemical reactions down the spinal cord to the nerves of the penis. A 2004 article in the *New York Times* concentrated on the important role of one section of the brain, the amygdale, on sexual activity; the article was entitled "The Biggest Sexual Organ is the Brain." "Messenger" chemicals stimulated by the brain cause an increase in the amount of blood entering large cavernous areas in the muscles of the penis and decrease the flow of blood away from the penis. The resultant increased pressure of the blood in the penis is mediated through the penile muscles and causes an erection. The final chemical reaction in this complex process is affected by an enzyme known as PDE-5 (phosphodiesterase). If this enzyme is inhibited there is an increased effect of an important chemical (cyclic guanosine monophophospate) on the erectile process. Don't get panicked by the scientific jargon. There is a very practical outcome. It was discovered that certain drugs act as PDE-5 inhibitors, and help a sexually excited man achieve improved penile rigidity. These include Viagra, Cialis and Levitra, which are household words, even though phosphodiesterase isn't, although that's where it all started.

Any abnormalities which involve circulation, the nervous system from the brain on down, including psychological factors, diminished muscular function and hormonal/chemical disorders can lead to erectile dysfunction. Many drugs, including those used to treat high blood pressure and psychiatric disorders also can adversely affect sexual function. The classic example is diabetes, in which there is often poor circulatory and nerve function. The treatment is to control the diabetes, as well as to try PDE-5 inhibitors.

This outline is an oversimplification of the complex factors involved in normal sexual activity. The complicated, multisystem causes of erectile dysfunction explain why many disorders can adversely affect sexual performance. It is generally agreed that, aside from the changes of aging, the commonest causes of erectile dysfunction are psychological and emotional in nature. We have all heard of the case in which a man has erectile dysfunction when sleeping with his wife, but not when cheating on her. The subject of sex is filled with folklore, myths and, of course, relevant humor. Like the one about the man who goes to the doctor with the complaint that "My sex urge is too high." Although the doctor felt this was an unusual complaint he performed a thorough examination and ordered a series of tests. He then told the patient: "All the results are normal. It's all in your mind." The reply was: "I know it's all in my mind. That's too high! I want you to bring it down!' The message is that if you have erectile dysfunction, absence of the foreskin is the unlikeliest of causes and the least of your worries.

10

Circumcision and the Military

A number of years ago a close friend of mine, on the occasion of his 65th birthday, was reminiscing about some of his experiences early in life, and he related an unusual situation that he faced in 1944, at the age of 18, shortly after joining the U.S. Navy. As an inductee he was sent to the San Diego Naval Base for basic training, "boot camp." He was issued uniforms, assigned to a platoon, and sent to the barracks. Shortly after moving in, the platoon was asked to line up, and the petty officer in charge asked: "Are there any Jews in this group?" My friend was shocked. He thought that Hitler might have won the war and, as a Jew, he was going to be sent to a concentration camp. He stepped forward along with other Jewish sailors. Far from being interned, this group was told to go to the recreation area, enjoy themselves and report back to the barracks in an hour. The other inductees were told to drop their pants in preparation for an inspection of their genitals by a navy medic, a "short arm inspection." The medic went down the line checking the circumcision status of the young men (even in the 1940s most U.S. males had been circumcised), and asking the uncircumcised men to retract the foreskin. Those with an unretractable or tight foreskin were sent to the infirmary to be circumcised. In those days (it might still be the same today, as it was in the 1950s when

I was in the Navy) the armed forces had their own brand of "informed consent." They informed, you consented. After a few days the selected men returned to the barracks with sore, circumcised penises and completed boot camp with the rest. As for my friend, he said it was one of the few times in his life when he felt that being a Jew put him in a privileged position, and he was happy not to be one of the "chosen" people to be circumcised as an adult, and grateful at having been circumcised at age 8 days.

They used to say that an army moves on its stomach. Admittedly, proper nutrition is important, but there are other non-military factors that are key to the success of armed forces. In earlier days more soldiers died from diseases and the elements than from battle. Think of Napoleon's troops in the invasion of Russia. Less than 10% of the invading forces returned, and the main causes for the decimation of the French army were the cold and deadly diseases such as typhoid, typhus, pneumonia, and cholera. In the carnage of our Civil War almost 600,000 young men died, slightly less than 400,000 among the Union troops and 200,000 Confederate soldiers. Two thirds of the Union soldiers and three fourths of the Confederates died of non-combat causes.

World War II was the first great armed conflict in which more soldiers died in battle than from disease. Modern military forces are well supplied with food, protected against the elements, immunized against many infectious diseases, and have antibiotics available to treat others. But there are still medical conditions which can take a soldier away from duty and thus preclude the fighting effectiveness of an army. The armed forces are made up of young men at the peak of sexual desire, frequently far away from home, without an available outlet for their feelings. To fill this sexual void, red light districts spring up wherever there are army camps or navy harbors. And where there are prostitutes there are sexually transmitted diseases (STDs). Also, wars are often fought in inhospitable places such as deserts and jungles, where adequate hygiene is a problem. When we talk about STDs and genital hygiene we talk about circumcision. Isn't it a stretch to think that circumcision can play a role in the availability of soldiers for combat? Not according to the experiences of the U.S. Army in World War II.

What was the basis for the armed forces circumcising young men before sending them off to war? It couldn't be the decision of sadistic officers to test young men for reaction to stress. This is America. There must have been good medical reasons for prophylactic circumcisions which were relevant to military service. There were. The answers can be found in one of a remarkable series of books published by the Medical Department of the U.S. Army entitled *Surgery in World War II*. The data relating to circumcision are found in the volume on Urology.

During the invasion of North Africa, in the early days of our involvement in the war, the U.S. Army was in the desert, fighting alongside the British, in the campaign against the German armies led by General Rommel, The Desert Fox. The situation was oppressive. It was hot, with lots of sand and little water. There was barely enough water for drinking, let alone washing, and hygiene was poor. In an uncircumcised man, sand and dirt were trapped under the foreskin. This led to infection of the penis with attendant swelling and inability to retract the foreskin, conditions known as balanoposthitis, phimosis and paraphimosis. Balanoposthitis is infection of the head of the penis (glans) and the inner layer of the foreskin. It causes pain and swelling, and there is often a foul-smelling discharge. Phimosis is inability to retract the foreskin, due to narrowing of the opening at the tip of the penis. In paraphimosis the foreskin can be retracted with difficulty, but due to swelling it cannot be pushed back and it traps the head of the penis, leading to severe pain and increased swelling. Another condition, condylomas, known as venereal warts, is seen more commonly on and under the foreskin. During the period from 1942-1945 these 4 conditions, associated with uncircumcised men—balanoposthitis, phimosis, paraphimosis, and condylomas—accounted for a total of 146,793 hospital admissions among U.S. servicemen in North Africa and Europe. It was realized that the man-hours lost as a result of these hospitalizations were costly to the war effort. In many instances it was necessary to treat the conditions with circumcision, whether immediately, or after the acute infection subsided, in order to prevent recurrences. The sheer numbers of soldiers unavailable for combat because of foreskin-related disorders was frustrating to commanding officers. It was stated that: "Higher headquarters sometimes questioned the number of circumcisions performed in the theater with an emphasis on days lost from duty. But all were performed from medical necessity." In referring to the almost 150,000 admissions related to the foreskin the army urologists stated that "Had these patients been circumcised before induction, this total would probably have been close to zero." Such experiences, beginning early in the war, offer an explanation for the circumcisions performed on young recruits in boot camp in 1944, and for the lasting impression on my friend in his reminiscences 47 years later.

The North African campaign also provided evidence for the relationship of the foreskin to a sexually transmitted disease (STD), chancroid, which is characterized by an infected sore on the head of the penis, usually beneath the foreskin. During an 8 month period in 1944, 7,318 cases of chancroid were seen at an Army venereal disease center in Naples. Surgical drainage or circumcision was often necessary in these cases. Of 1,000 circumcisions performed at the center during that time, about half were done to treat chancroid. The increased prevalence of chancroid in uncircumcised men was later confirmed during the Korean War, in 1950-52, when it was found that 90% of the cases of chancroid occurred in uncircumcised men, who made up only about 30% of the troops.

Servicemen returning from World War II had become aware of the medical advantages of circumcision, and as they became fathers, the newborn circumcision rate in the United States rose to a reported peak level of 85-90% in the 1950s. This circumcision rate fell in the early 1970s with concern about any procedures leading to discomfort in the newborn period, as well as through an ill-advised anti-circumcision policy of the American Academy of Pediatrics (AAP), which will be discussed later. The past and current rate of circumcision in the U.S. will be addressed in the section on statistics (Chapter 13)

The military's interest in the advantages of circumcision was rekindled in the Gulf War, when the problems of sand and hygiene again led to local penile disorders in uncircumcised soldiers.

With regard to sexually transmitted diseases (STDs) and circumcision, the relationship was supported by a report from the Canadian Army in 1947, which was based on World War II experiences. The author, Dr. R.A Wilson, presented evidence that both syphilis and gonorrhea, but particularly syphilis, are more likely to occur in uncircumcised men. He offered medical explanations. In the case of gonorrhea it was felt that the warmth and moisture of the area under the foreskin was an ideal environment, allowing for multiplication of the bacteria which could then contaminate the urethra, causing local infection with the typical thick, yellow discharge. For syphilis, which spreads throughout the body, the portal of entry for the spirochete into the bloodstream was considered to be the multiple small abrasions and tears of the delicate foreskin membrane that occur during intercourse. In 1988, more than 40 years later, a Canadian epidemiologist, Dr. Stephen Moses, analyzed multiple studies relating

STDs to circumcision status. The evidence was overwhelming in favor of the role of the foreskin in increasing the risk of acquiring syphilis and chancroid, with 11 major studies all showing a protective effect of circumcision. The evidence of predisposition to gonorrhea was strong but not as powerful; in 7 large series, 5 studies showed a protective effect of circumcision and in 2 no effect was seen.

So, from the standpoint of current armed forces, the presence of the foreskin in a soldier increases the risk of local penile problems (balanoposthitis, phimosis and paraphimosis) as well as certain STDs (syphilis, chancroid, and probably gonorrhea), all of which can result in loss of availability of troops for combat. This risk of the foreskin is particularly high in regions where adequate hygiene is unavailable, including deserts, jungles and rugged mountainous areas, just the places where modern battles are being fought.

As for the most dangerous STD of all, that due to the human immunodeficiency virus (HIV), at this time it is of limited interest to the military. This is in spite of the fact that tens of millions of people worldwide have died from the disease, and the AIDS epidemic is spreading. As we have discussed, the foreskin has been shown to be an important risk factor in acquiring HIV infection, due to the role of special cells that bind the virus, as well as the presence of mini-abrasions and tears that allow HIV to enter the system. But the AIDS epidemic is occurring in underdeveloped parts of the world, mainly in sub-Saharan Africa, and, to a lesser extent in Asia. This is of limited interest to the world's greatest military power, the U.S. Armed Forces. I would predict that if large sections of the U.S. Army were to be dispatched to sub-Saharan Africa, a lot more attention would be given to making sure all men were circumcised.

PART II: CONSEQUENCES

11

Non-Science, Nonsense, Quotes and Anecdotes

The organized, activist lay anti-circumcision movement began in the late 1960's and early 1970's. It was a time when non-intervention, "natural" care and "infant bonding" were being promoted. In 1971 the American Academy of Pediatrics (AAP) issued a statement that "there is no valid medical indication for newborn circumcision." Many groups opposed to circumcision were formed, each with a different emphasis and membership, and all with picturesque acronyms. The world epicenter of the anti-circumcision movement was and is in the San Francisco Bay area. Here's a real life example.

Adam London was a healthy, normal-developing toddler when his mother brought charges against the physician who performed Adam's newborn circumcision, as well as the medical organization with which the physician was associated. The details of this case were reported in 1985 in the *Marin Independent Journal*, a well known Northern California newspaper. What was the complaint of the plaintiff? Was the doctor inexperienced and unqualified to perform circumcision? No, he had practiced for years and done many circumcisions. Had the doctor botched the circumcision causing damage to the penis through negligence, and was he being sued for malpractice? No, the circumcision was routine, and the penis looked fine. Was there failure to get informed consent? No, both parents had signed the informed consent form, although they were subsequently divorced, and the charges were being brought by the mother. Then what was the basis for the lawsuit and what were the charges? The mother claimed, with support from a well organized, activist anti-circumcision group called NOCIRC, that routine circumcision, even when performed competently by a fully qualified physician, causes permanent emotional damage to the baby boy, and is therefore criminal activity. The unsuspecting doctor was charged with battery, cruelty, false imprisonment, infliction of pain, child abuse, kidnapping and mayhem. If convicted the physician could have faced life in prison for simply performing an uncomplicated circumcision. One would think that these bizarre allegations would immediately be discredited and thrown out of court, and fortunately they were. In dismissing the charges the judge affirmed a legal fact which seems to be obvious. Parents have the right to consent for their infant or minor child to have medical procedures, such as immunizations or circumcision, which have preventive health benefits. The intimidating tactics in the London case are characteristic of the organized, activist lay anti-circumcision groups. They try to use any methods to further their cause, whether it is through using a stick, as in this case in Marin County, California, or by offering a carrot, as was done with the Royal Family of England.

After the birth of their second son, Prince Charles and Princess Diana were no doubt surprised to learn that they had been chosen Parents of the Year by the above-mentioned NOCIRC. It seems that since the time of Queen Victoria all males of the British Royal Family were circumcised shortly after birth. In keeping with this tradition the circumcision of the infant Prince Charles was carried out in Buckingham Palace by Dr. Jacob Snowman, a well known London physician, who was not only a surgeon, but an Orthodox Jew and a Mohel, a religious circumciser. But the new Royal young couple decided to end this traditional circumcision practice and both of their sons, the Princes William and Harry, were left "intact," the word used by the opponents of circumcision to describe the uncircumcised state. The reasons for this decision are not clear. The National Health Service had decided, for economic reasons, to stop paying for routine newborn circumcision, and as a result the circumcision rate in the United Kingdom was falling. At the same time it had become fashionable to try avoiding all discomfort to newborns. Babies were being born as soft music played, and they were placed into warm water to ease the transition from the womb to the harsh outside world. Princess Diana was a modern woman, very attuned to style, and she could have been influenced by the fact that the uncircumcised penis was beginning to be considered "genital chic." I don't know whether the Prince and Princess ever took note of their NOCIRC honor.

In condemning newborn male circumcision, the anti-circumcision movement has attempted to equate it with a primitive ritualistic act in young girls called "female circumcision," which has been banned in many countries. Male circumcision ("cutting around") as has been described, is a simple operation to remove the foreskin, and it has many proven medical benefits. "Female circumcision," on the other hand, is a much more extensive procedure with no known medical benefits. As generally performed, it consists of complete removal of the clitoris and the labia, with the borders of the labia being sewed together, to make a very small, tight vaginal opening, presumably to prevent early intercourse. The anatomical equivalent in the male would be to cut off the entire penis, as well as the skin that covers the testicles (the scrotum). Comparing male circumcision to female genital mutilation is like equating a "nose job" (rhinoplasty) to a decapitation.

How much effect has the proliferation of anti-circumcision organizations in the past 20-25 years had on the circumcision rate in the U.S.? Surprisingly, almost none. According to the statistics of the Center for Disease Control (CDC) and the National Center for Health Statistics (NCHS) in the 20 year period from 1979-1999 the U.S. newborn male circumcision rate went from 64.3% to 65.3%, no overall change. We will discuss the statistics of newborn circumcision in the U.S. in Chapter 13. Anti-circumcision groups have had a small measure of success with some "trendy" middle class parents and dissatisfied men in a few conclaves, mainly on the West Coast (Berkeley, Marin County, parts of Los Angeles) and in the East (New York suburbs).

Since the anti-circumcision groups have been unsuccessful in decreasing circumcision among the general public in the U.S. they have turned their frustration and desperation into an attack on the most vulnerable and defenseless part of the population– poor children. Parents on welfare have no political or economic power, and are at the mercy of State bureaucracies and legislatures for decisions on the medical care of their children. Knowing this, 22 anti-circumcision groups have banded together and formed a lobbying organization—the International Coalition of Genital Integrity (ICGI)—which has been pressuring State legislatures to eliminate coverage for newborn circumcision to Medicaid recipients. The argument that eliminating payment for newborn circumcision would save money has resonated with legislative bodies faced with increasing budgetary deficits. This callous, insensitive activism has been successful, and 13 states now refuse to pay for newborn circumcision for welfare recipients regardless of the parent's wishes. These include Arizona,

California, Florida, Maine, Mississippi, Missouri, Montana, Nevada, North Carolina, North Dakota, Oregon, Utah and Washington.

Some have spoken out against this disregard of the wishes of poor parents. An editorial in the St. Petersburg Times criticized Florida legislators who "never stop boasting about an agenda they say promotes families and "more personal freedom." Then they halt Medicaid coverage for newborn circumcision—a surgical procedure that the nation's most respected medical professionals say should be a decision left to families and their doctors." In quoting one state legislator who said that halting funding for circumcision was a "no-brainer" the editorial went on to say: "This is a terrible message—that poor people don't deserve the right to make a medical, cultural and religious choice that is available to everyone else." So much for the claim of the anti-circumcision groups that they are out to protect the rights of the child.

With the great majority of mainstream, middle class boys in the U.S. being circumcised, an uncircumcised boy in this country is marked as either an immigrant, a son of recent immigrants or a child of poverty (with the exception of a few middle class followers of the anti-circ movement). To cope with this social disadvantage of the foreskin, some poor parents, sadly and courageously, have scraped together enough money to pay for newborn circumcision from their meager assets, in order to give their sons the appearance of mainstream American boys. The cost of newborn circumcision for middle class boys is covered by health insurance, but in 13 states poor parents will have to raise the money themselves if they want their sons circumcised.

The anti-circumcision groups have argued unsuccessfully that by agreeing to have their newborn sons circumcised, parents are robbing the infants of their human rights. In a brazen example of hypocrisy apparently they feel that newborns should have the right to choose or refuse circumcision, but not poor people. The opponents of circumcision have met with some success in punishing the weak and helpless, but have had no effect on the general American public.

Over the past years I have received many personal communications and seen more on the Internet expressing various opinions, often contradictory, on the topic of circumcision. Here are some examples:

It Brings Up Questions

"Dear Wendy: My husband and I are expecting our first son and have decided not to circumcise him. I think the practice is barbaric: my husband is swayed by the recent medical literature. How do we break the news to our parents?" (Question to the "Ask Wendy" column of the Jewish newspaper, *The Forward,* 2001.)(Possible answer: "Cautiously, particularly if your parents are observant Jews and are helping you buy a house.")

"My husband of many years recently expressed his feelings of anger and loss at the fact that he was circumcised as a baby. More recently he told me he had found some information on the Internet about foreskin restoration which involves taping and stretching the remaining skin to form a kind of substitute foreskin. He has started to do that. Is this a sign of male menopause or what? As far as I can determine he has very adequate sensitivity and has never experienced any kind of problem that I am aware of. Furthermore I don't particularly care for the appearance of uncircumcised penises." Question sent to the "Sex Matters" column of the *San Francisco Examiner,* Oct. 17, 1997. (Possible answer: "You make a very good case for male menopause. On the bright side a trophy foreskin is probable better than a trophy lover.")

It Can Have Surprising Effects

"I just disagree with your devaluing of the foreskin. Despite its extra hygiene requirements and attendant risks it provides pleasure and protects from frostbite." Personal Internet message to me, 2001

"At age 40 years I decided to have circumcision done because it was almost impossible to keep down odor and discomfort. Once done a whole new freedom from above, cleanliness is so easy now. (And I believe ladies like it so).Also I can stand the heat better now." Personal handwritten letter, 1997

It's a Bad Thing

"I am 24 and was circumcised at birth. I only recently had a sudden increase of rage and bitterness at the thought of being circumcised." NOCIRC Newsletter.
I was circumcised on day 7 and suffered post traumatic syndrome ever since my earliest awareness." *NOCIRC Newsletter,* 1994.

"I believe that at least part of the reason why I have not been hired at the University of Washington is because I have been circumcised." Personal correspondence, August 1992.

Many other examples of alleged unfavorable effects of circumcision can be found on the Internet. The following quotes are from the other side of the coin.

It's a Good Thing

"Indeed improved sexual satisfaction for male and female may be more beneficial than the usually given medical reasons for circumcision. My own circumcision as an adult indicates that this is true." Dr Valentine, pen name for a physician, *Medical Aspects of Human Sexuality*, 1974.

"We chose to have our son circumcised because we have family members and friends that weren't and now wish they had been." Internet message 2003.

"I had my 2 sons circumcised for a number of reasons, including- 1. Cleanliness- an uncircumcised penis is not inherently dirty, but boys don't tend to clean too carefully – just look under their fingernails, 2. I heard from a urologist's wife that he frequently gets requests from teenagers and men who weren't circumcised as infants and want to be circumcised. That cinched it for me. Easier done as a baby than as an adult." Internet communication 2003.

I definitely urge parents to circumcise their boys as infants. There's no reason to have to go through all the trouble that I've been through." Recently circumcised man, Internet communication, 2001.

"I am a mother of a very happy circumcised 3 ½ year old boy. One mother has posted a web site showing step by step of a newborn being circumcised. I find this horribly distasteful! When my son was circumcised the procedure was totally painless and non-traumatic." Internet communication, 2001.

"I don't want my son having a penis that looks like a dog's." Comment by the father of recently circumcised baby as the reason he chose circumcision. 2002.

"I think it is wrong for parents to purposely make their sons unusual (in this country—USA) by leaving a foreskin on their sons' penises. They might as well tattoo the word "Odd" on their foreheads." Posted on the Internet 1999 by "Denny."

"I've been in nursing for 10 years and every uncircumcised patient I've had has had problems when they were older, and when they were younger, they smelled." Internet correspondence, 1997.

"As a man who is glad to have been circumcised at birth, I can honestly say I have had no problems or regrets, and would unreservedly recommend any friend to have their child circumcised. I have been dismayed to discover that the net has become an instrument of propaganda for a position that does not correspond to my experience." Internet correspondence, 1997.

Foreskin Restorationists

At the extreme end of the anti-circumcision spectrum are those men who would like to replace their missing foreskin. Here are some opinions from this group:

"Chris has been "restoring" his foreskin. Stretching it, really. He used an elastic band that ran down his leg, swinging once around his knee and clipping to his sock. At night he clips the elastic around his shoulder to pull on him more while he sleeps. It wasn't a project at all. It was a cause. He was reasserting the rights of his gender – to remain intact, to obtain sexual pleasure, to not get cut." From "The Foreskin Saga" by John Sedgwick, *GQ* magazine, Feb. 2000.

"Al Parker, self-described porn king, recently underwent a surgical foreskin restoration, when he spoke to The Advocate. Parker jokes about the procedure which cost him $5000. Now that he has his penis the way he wants it, Parker can get on with his film career. The new foreskin will debut in the upcoming "Al Parker, the Uncut Version," which is scheduled for a 1990 release." From an article entitled "May the Foreskin Be With You" by Christopher Michaud, in *The Advocate* magazine, 1989. (Haven't seen any reviews—guess the foreskin debut was disappointing).

"Custom-made devices are now available, the most popular being "the Tugger," formerly the Penis Uncircumcising Device (PUD).It retails at $115 plus shipping and handling. Richard DeSeabra, head of the New York chapter of NORM (National Organization of Restoring Males) was running in the subway once when the device became undone and a small weighted ball flew out of his pants. "Sometimes I'll be at work and one of the weights will clank up against the desk and everybody will say, 'What the hell is that?'" From "Unkindest Cut" by Stephen Rodrick, *New Republic* magazine, May 29, 1995.

In listening to testimonials and anecdotes from the public it is apparent that circumcision is good, circumcision is bad, circumcision improves sex, and circumcision hinders sex. The foreskin is the center for sexual pleasure, the foreskin gets in the way of sexual pleasure, the foreskin is a harbinger of dirt and bacteria, and the foreskin is self-cleaning. Removing the foreskin opens up new vistas of cleanliness and health, trying to replace an absent foreskin or stretch what is left can change one's life. There are physicians who compare circumcision to removal of the breasts, vulva, eyelids, all the teeth and one testicle, in spite of the fact that they presumably understand anatomy and organ functions. The message is that pro and con anecdotes and testimonials cancel each other out. The answer is that one must look to responsible clinical research which is on firm scientific ground and is published in peer-reviewed medical journals. This objective information has steadily accumulated over the past 100 years, particularly in the past 2 decades, and it overwhelmingly favors the medical advantages of newborn circumcision.

Circumcision, being controversial and having a prurient aspect, has spawned a good deal of media interest. "The big issue over a little tissue" is how *Penthouse* magazine characterized the circumcision controversy in a 1993 article entitled: "The Penis Page. Facts and Phalluses of America's Favorite Organ." The title set the tone for the message, which, surprisingly, presented both sides of the question. The author predicted a big battle, presumably launched by anti-circumcision forces, "when the Clinton health plan comes out in favor of routine circumcision," Well, we all know the fate of the Clinton health plan, and the big battle has been downgraded to periodic skirmishes promoted by organized circumcision opposition groups. Those favoring circumcision claim the factual high ground if they can get a hearing in order to present the convincing evidence of the multiple health benefits of newborn circumcision. Circumcision opponents dominate the Internet with multiple websites, concentrating on anecdotes and testimonials.

My personal experience with the media began in 1987, when I was appointed Chair of the American Academy of Pediatrics Task Force on Circumcision. I had no idea what I was in for when I became involved in the circumcision issue. The emotions ran high, and I was immediately in the sights of the anti- circumcision groups, who wanted their agenda to become the official AAP policy. Since our 1989 AAP report on circumcision I have been interviewed by magazines and newspapers, and have appeared on radio and television, often with an anti-circumcision representative.

Among the programs that have featured circumcision are *20/20*, *Nightline* and the Joan Rivers, Nachman and Phil Donahue shows to name a few. In most instances the guests and messages have been opposed to circumcision.

The picture has been pretty much the same with newspapers and magazines. Most of the articles have an anti-circumcision slant. Of special interest is the coverage in the Jewish print media, where there has been a lot of attention devoted to a recent phenomenon, the refusal of some Jewish parents to have their infant sons circumcised. And this is not only in American Jews. An article in the *Jerusalem Post* referred to the practice of a few secular Israeli Jews of leaving their sons uncircumcised.

Similarly, the circumcision sites on the Internet are predominantly anti-circumcision, consisting largely of anecdotes, testimonials and unsubstantiated opinions. If one types in the word "circumcision," very few of the many sites that come up have objective information or favor the procedure.

The continued high circumcision rate in the U.S in the face of a generally anti-circumcision media attests to the commitment of the public to this procedure. This is illustrated by an interview with a young couple on a Discovery Channel program in 2000. The woman stated that she was satisfied with sex with her uncircumcised boyfriend "who is very clean," but that if she had a son she would have him circumcised, "because I'm an American." In this country circumcision has almost become a form of patriotism.

12

American Academy of Pediatrics—
Not Its Finest Hour

"There are no valid medical indications for circumcision in the neonatal period." These 12 words with minor variations were destined to become the official policy of the American Academy of Pediatrics (AAP) for a period of almost 20 years. The single, undocumented sentence first appeared in 1971 in a publication of the AAP Committee on the Fetus and Newborn entitled "Hospital Care of Newborn Infants." The only reference cited was to an anti-circumcision article, "Whither the Foreskin?" No explanation or evidence was offered by the anonymous author of the statement, but it had a profound effect. It became the rallying cry and the rationale for the formation and growth of a rising number of lay anti-circumcision organizations, which previously had been considered to be over-the-line fringe groups. Opposition to newborn circumcision could now be said to be supported by the AAP, the respected specialty organization of the nation's children's doctors.

What was the basis for this "no valid indications" statement? One would expect that if a respected professional organization like the AAP issues an important clinical conclusion it is based on documented facts. This could be in the form of important published studies in the medical literature or data collected by the organization itself. At the time, in

1971, over 80% of newborn boys in the U.S. were being circumcised. Reversing this practice would represent a major
shift in routine newborn care. Yet, no evidence was given to
justify a change. Even more disturbing, it seemed as if the
author(s) were unaware of the many published studies indicating that there were indeed medical benefits of newborn
circumcision. Those of you who have read the first half of
this book know the medical evidence and proven advantages.
By 1971 there had been 3 major publications in leading journals, all showing that invasive, lethal penile cancer is a disease almost never found in circumcised men. The experiences of the Armed Forces in World War II had been published,
showing that over 145,000 uncircumcised soldiers were tem-
porarily lost to duty due to foreskin-related problems. The
Canadian armed services report, almost 20 years earlier,
showed that uncircumcised men were more likely than were
circumcised men to acquire sexually transmitted diseases,
particularly syphilis. And then there is phimosis and balanoposthitis, most cases of which occur in childhood. How
could anyone make a statement about circumcision without
mentioning this considerable evidence? The answer, in my
mind, is that the originator of the 'no valid indications" sentence was unaware of the previous data, and uninterested in
looking for any circumcision benefits that might accrue after
the newborn period. I believe the basic problem was territo-
rial-the decision was being made in the wrong jurisdiction by
a professional group with an anti-circumcision bias, the AAP
Committee of the Fetus and Newborn.

The AAP Committee on the Fetus and Newborn is made up
mainly of neonatologists, specialists in newborn medicine, usually hospital-based. They work in Newborn Intensive Care Units
on desperately sick infants, including those with serious diseases
and severe prematurity. They are dedicated to saving lives and preventing the ravages of immaturity and life-threatening diseases in

newborns, and resistant to any activity which takes them away from this task. Most neonatologists I have known have less interest in full term healthy newborns than they do in sick and premature babies. They almost never will have contact with a normal infant after he/she leaves the hospital nursery and goes home. Newborn circumcision violates their frame of reference in 2 ways. First of all, it is an elective procedure which utilizes nursery space and personnel, and can result in delayed discharge if the infant needs observation after the procedure. It distracts them from the care of sick infants. Secondly, since elective circumcision, like immunizations, is a preventive health measure, the benefits accrue later in infancy, childhood and adult life. A neonatologist can function as an outstanding professional in spite of having no interest in or knowledge of phimosis, balanoposthitis, or post-discharge urinary tract infection in infants and children, let alone sexually transmitted diseases and penile cancer in adults. With the exception of Dr. Tom Wiswell, who was Chief of Neonatology at Walter Reed Armed Forces Hospital when he observed the predominance of infant kidney infections in uncircumcised infant boys, I cannot recall knowing any neonatologist who was in favor of newborn circumcision. For a neonatologist, an anti-circumcision viewpoint comes with the territory. Even Dr. Wiswell, prior to his pioneering discovery, had written in opposition to newborn circumcision. Placing the decision on newborn circumcision in the hand of a committee of neonatologists is putting the foxes in charge of the chicken coop. There is no evidence that the neonatologists were knowingly given such a charge by the AAP. I think it is more likely that the anonymous author of the single undocumented sentence, "no valid medical indications" etc, just wrote it from the top of his/her head, and placed it in the newborn booklet. From there it was picked up by the lay anti-circumcision groups, got carried away, and it's still with us in varying forms.

The concern of pediatricians with the lack of documen-

tation of the 1971 statement led to a decision by the AAP
to revisit the issue of circumcision in 1975, this time with a
4-member Ad Hoc Task Force on Circumcision. The Task
Force consisted of a neonatologist, an obstetrician, an urologist, and a respected general pediatrician, Dr. Hugh Thompson was Chairman. After reviewing the data in the literature,
it was apparent that there were medical benefits of circumcision that were "valid," including prevention of penile cancer,
avoidance of local foreskin disorders and ease of genital hygiene. It would seem that the logical conclusion would simply be to state these facts, admit that a mistake was made
and reverse the erroneous 1971 statement. The problem was
that the 1975 Circumcision Task Force was responsible to the
AAP Committee on the Fetus and Newborn, which had issued the original flawed statement. It was decided that rather
than reverse the original policy and own up to the mistake,
creative verbiage should be used. The new conclusion stated that "there is no absolute medical indication for routine
circumcision of the newborn." Since there are few, if any,
absolutes in the world, the statement was safe, but misleading and a misrepresentation of the facts. The 1975 Circumcision Task Force Chairman, Dr. Thompson, was upset by
this sleight-of-hand word change and in 1983 when the 1975
"no absolute indication" statement was reiterated by both
the AAP and the Obstetric group (ACOG), he expressed his
frustration in an editorial in the *American Journal of Diseases of Childhood,* but there was not much he could do.
When I called him in 1987, after my appointment as Chair
of a new Task Force on Circumcision, he was still resentful.
By allowing the Committee on the Fetus and Newborn to remain in charge of circumcision policy, the AAP had abridged
its responsibility. Not only had the foxes been put in charge
of the chicken coop, but when chickens started to disappear,
the investigation was handed over to a delegation of foxes.

The conclusion, not surprisingly, was that there was "no absolute indication" that chickens were the only source of food for foxes. The 1975 "no absolute medical indication" statement remained the official policy of the AAP until the 1989 report of the next Task Force on Circumcision, of which I was Chair.

The stimulus for the appointment of a new Task Force in 1987 was the "Wiswell Report," a large study using the Armed Forces data base, which totaled over 200,000 newborn boys, and found that uncircumcised male infants in the first year of life were 10-20 times more likely to get kidney infection as were circumcised boys. My co- members of the Task Force included an urologist (Dr. Frank Hinman, a well known senior Professor of Urology in San Francisco), an obstetrician (Dr. Constance Bohon of Washington, D.C.), a pediatric surgeon (Dr. Glen Anderson, Minneapolis, MN), a general pediatrician (Dr. E. Maurice Wakeman from Guilford, CT), and a neonatologist, Dr. Ronald Poland, who was Chairman of the Committee on the Fetus and Newborn of the AAP. Our Task Force had a consultant, Dr. David Minenberg, a well known pediatric urologist from New York City, who was head of the Section of Urology of the AAP. The Task Force was appointed in December 1987, and the next month nine specific topics were split up and assigned to individual Task Force members; cancer of the penis, cervical cancer of the uterus, sexually transmitted diseases, urinary tract infections, pain and psychological effects, surgical techniques, complications, local penile problems and ease of hygiene, and surgical complications. The members were instructed to research these topics and develop a reference list. Having a bibliography was considered important to foster credibility of the conclusions, since neither the 1971 nor 1975 reports had references, except for the anti-circumcision opinion piece referred to in 1971. We didn't want to make the mistakes of these 2 earlier reports, which simply represented the un-documented feelings and opinions of physicians with varying degrees of expertise on the subject. We met in Chicago on March 18, 1988, collated the results of our individual inves-tigations, and I had the task of combining all the collected information into a final report. It turned out the Task Force was a very cooperative and compatible group, although it was apparent that Dr. Poland as head of the AAP Committee on the Fetus and Newborn was very resistant to changing the negative conclusions of the earlier reports of that committee. After a series of phone conferences and additional research, a final report was ready in June 1988, and submitted to the Executive Board of the AAP. We expected rapid approval, and underestimated the bureaucracy of the AAP, but final-ly, after a delay of 5 months, our report was released and published in the official AAP journal, *Pediatrics,* in August 1989. Most importantly the negative statements of 1971 and 1975 were reversed. We found that, although there are disad-vantages and risks to newborn circumcision, the procedure results in medical benefits. Local penile problems—phimo-sis, paraphimosis, and balanoposthitis—are prevented. The incidence of penile cancer is decreased. Infant urinary tract infections may be decreased, but more confirmatory stud-ies were needed. Cancer of the cervix had been found to be more likely in sexual partners of uncircumcised men infected with human papilloma virus. The earliest reports had been published suggesting that circumcised men were less likely to acquire HIV infection, but we were urged to stay away from that explosive issue until there was more evidence, and we did. We concluded that the benefits and risks of newborn circumcision should be objectively explained to the parents and informed consent obtained. The role of physician was to engage in "non-directional counseling," empowering the parents with documented information, rather than assuming a "doctor knows best" attitude. The response to our 1989 report was variable. The anti-circumcision forces were predictably devastated by the reversal of the previous negative position of the AAP. Parents electing circumcision of their newborn sons felt that the medical evidence justified their decision. But the press would have preferred a more definitive decision, looking upon our conclusions as being neutral. We felt that the final confirmatory evidence for disorders such as kidney infection, HIV and cervical cancer would be apparent within a few years. In addition, further experience would determine the safety of local anesthesia for pain relief.

In the 10 years between the release of our report in 1989, and the appointment of a new Task Force on Circumcision in 1999, a large body of evidence accumulated confirming and extending the benefits of newborn circumcision which we had documented earlier. Wiswell's original findings of infant urinary infection were supported by 12 separate studies from around the world, showing an average of tenfold protection by circumcision. Over 20 additional studies, mainly from sub-Saharan Africa, had found that uncircumcised men were 2-7 times more likely to acquire HIV following sexual exposure. And pain, one of the troublesome disadvantages of newborn circumcision, was demonstrated to be effectively and safely eliminated by the use of local anesthesia. With accumulated proof of more advantages and less disadvantages one would have predicted that the AAP would clearly state that the benefits of newborn circumcision clearly exceeded the risks. But don't bet on it.

The 1997-99 Task Force on Circumcision was headed by Dr. Carole Lannon, an epidemiologist (specialist in statistics and public health) from North Carolina, and included members from the fields of anesthesia, infectious disease, urology, neonatology, obstetrics and general pediatrics. They planned to use an "evidence-based approach," which was commendable in view of the published data that had accrued since the time of our report in 1989. This new evidence reinforced the benefits we thought were tentative and addressed the issue of pain by demonstrating the effectiveness and safety of local anesthesia. But unexplainably, when the new report came out in 1999, more benefits of circumcision had been magically transformed into less reason to circumcise. Positive evidence had been converted into a negative statement. Although potential benefits were recognized and referenced, they were downgraded throughout the report, and the final conclusion was that "these data are not sufficient to recommend routine neonatal circumcision." No explanation was given, and there was no hint as to how much evidence if any would be "sufficient" to convince this group. No attempt was made to describe the benefits to risk ratio—listing the benefits in one column and the risks in the other. At least 6 benefits were described in the body of the report, including a protective effect of circumcision against penile cancer, infant urinary tract infections, HIV and syphilis, phimosis, paraphimosis and balanoposthitis. It also cited data which "suggests more varied sexual practice and less sexual dysfunction in circumcised adult men." To counterbalance these significant advantages of newborn circumcision, the 1999 AAP Task Force could come up with only one evidence-based disadvantage, the surgery complication rate. As with our report 10 years earlier it was found that the complication rate was low, 0.2-0.6%, and they stated that "most of the complications that do occur are minor." With 6 or more medical "benefits" and only one minor "risks" of newborn circumcision, this adds up to a benefits to risks ratio of 6 to 1. It is difficult to understand how the Task Force could have concluded their report with a negative viewpoint which discourages the procedure, and is a throwback to the 1971 (no valid indication) and 1975 (no absolute indication) statements. The only explanation that comes to mind is an anti-circumcision bias of the Chair and/or members which blinded the Task Force to the facts. Relevant is the possible role of Dr. Robert Van Howe, the outspoken anti-circumcision pediatrician from Wisconsin, who has referred to himself as "Consultant" to the 1999 Task Force. Although there is no official recognition that Dr. Van Howe was ever given this title, it appears that he did address the group, and there is a good deal of the jargon of the anti-circumcision organizations in the report (circumcision is referred to as "amputation of the foreskin").

When the report of the 1999 Task Force was released, those of us who have worked in the field and have knowledge of the evidence were incredulous. Dr. Tom Wiswell, who, in the mid-1980's performed the pioneering studies linking the foreskin to infant urinary tract infections, Dr. Stephen Moses, an epidemiologist who helped gather and analyze the data from Africa on HIV and circumcision, and I wrote a commentary for *Pediatrics,* the official journal of the AAP, which was published in 2000 as a Special Article ("New Policy on Circumcision—Cause for Concern"). We brought up many of the criticisms and discrepancies noted above. We pointed out one statement in the report that seemed to be irrelevant, if not bizarre. As a justification for not recommending newborn circumcision it was stated that the procedure is "not essential for the child's current well being." This misses the whole point of preventive pediatrics, a basic cornerstone in the care of children. The aim of newborn circumcision is not to affect the child's current well-being, but the FUTURE well-being, just as a polio injection is not given to treat the child today, but to prevent polio in the future. If all a pediatrician did was to treat the child's current problems, there would be no need for immunizations, preventive dentistry, or much of the counseling done by pediatricians. It is unbelievable to me that an AAP group, headed by an epidemiologist working in a Department of Community Medicine, wouldn't be aware of this basic role in pediatrics.

Understandably, the media interpreted the 1999 *Report of the AAP Task Force on Circumcision* as a step backwards. The wording of the conclusions had converted increased evidence favoring newborn circumcision into a statement opposing it. This was reflected in the headlines; "Pediatricians Turn Away from Circumcision" (CNN), "Circumcision Loses a Key Endorsement" (*Washington Post*)," Circumcision Benefits Disputed (*Chicago Sun Times*), and "Circumcision Opponents Energized by About Face of Academy of Pediatrics" (*Forward*). In one fell swoop the AAP had stepped back 30 years.

In the 5 years since the 1999 Task Force report, important data on the benefits of newborn circumcision have continued to accumulate, as described in Chapters 3-10.

Since the undocumented 1971 statement ("no valid indication") the AAP has mislead the public as well as physicians. In its pronouncements on newborn circumcision for over 30 years, the AAP has at best displayed disinterest and disregard of the evidence, and at worst demonstrated an anti-circumcision bias and misrepresentation of the facts. The good news is that neither the recommendations of the AAP nor the activism and media dominance of the anti-circumcision organizations have had much of an effect on American parents, a large majority of whom continue to choose circumcision for their newborn sons.

13

Circumcision Statistics—
Don't Believe Everything You Hear

When I traveled to New York City a few years ago to attend the 50th anniversary celebration of my medical school graduation, the experience was both uplifting and sobering. It was a pleasure to revisit the exciting early years of medical school during World War II, but the memorial list on the bulletin board of classmates who were no longer around was a reminder of our age and mortality. As my eyes ran down the list of our departed contemporaries, I was surprised to see the name of a friend to whom I had spoken a few minutes before. When I went back and pointed out to him his inclusion on the obituary list, his reply (with credit to Mark Twain) was: "The news of my demise is premature and exaggerated." Similarly, the opponents of newborn circumcision would have us believe that the procedure has been in failing health for over 20 years, is moribund, and within a few years will expire. Not so. Not only has newborn circumcision not decreased in the past 20 years, but it seems to be becoming more prevalent, with the exception of the sons of recent immigrants (mainly Hispanics). If one considers non-Hispanic males in the U.S., at least 75-80%, over 100 million Americans, are currently circumcised. Let's look at the facts, including the statistics from the U.S. government (the

Center for Disease Control (CDC) and the National Council
for Health Statistics (NCHS)), as well as published data from
private sources around the country.

The CDC/NCHS has published data covering the period
from 1979-1999, years when the claim was made that the
circumcision rate was falling. The figures show the percent
of newborn males with circumcision performed in short stay
hospitals where they were born. The data are broken down
by race and by 4 regions of the country (Midwest, Northeast,
South and West). There was no significant change in the percentage of U.S. infant boys being circumcised as newborns
in the hospital over this 20 year period. In 1979 64.3% of
newborns were being circumcised in the hospital before discharge, while in 1999 65.1% were circumcised. More revealing were the statistics from the 4 regions of the country. In
the Midwest the percentage of newborns circumcised rose
from 74.3% to 81.4% from 1979 to 1999, and in the South
from 55.6% to 64.1%. In the Northeast there was a slight
fall (from 66.2% to 65.4%). But in the West, particularly in
California, there was a marked fall in the rate of newborn
circumcision from 63.9% to 36.7%, with the rate falling
steadily over this 20 year period. What was the explanation
for the fall in percentage of circumcision done in newborn
hospitals in California, while in the rest of the country there
was either no change or a rise in circumcision rate? Does
it reflect the success of the anti-circumcision groups on the
West coast, where they are centered? Hardly. The reason for
the fall in circumcision in the West is the increasing births in
this region of infants of recent immigrants, mainly Hispanics, but also Asians, who are not circumcised for cultural
reasons. There has been a steady and rapid rise in Hispanic
births, so that by the turn of the 21st century over 50% of
newborn infants born in California were Hispanic and about
10% were Asians. Non-Hispanic white infants in California

now make up only about 30% of births. Even if 100% of non-Hispanic whites chose to have their newborn sons circumcised, the circumcision rate in the state would be less than 50%, assuming that fewer than 10% of Hispanic and Asian babies were circumcised. The primary role of immigrants in determining statistics in the West is demonstrated by the fact that over 80% of newborn boys are circumcised in the Midwest, the area of the country with the fewest immigrants, where non-Hispanic whites strongly predominate.

Non-governmental studies from around the country confirm the fact that, if non-immigrant births are not considered, the percentage of circumcised males in the United States is in the range of 80%. In Houston, Texas, 190 new middle class mothers were surveyed; 85% chose to have their newborn boys circumcised. Even though they had seen the American Academy of Pediatrics (AAP) brochure, they said this had no effect. The main reason for the decision was the circumcision status of the father. Higher parents' age and education were also associated with the decision to circumcise. At the opposite end of the country, in Atlanta, Georgia, almost 2000 hospital records from 1985 and 1986 were reviewed, revealing an 89% newborn circumcision rate in 1985 and 84% in 1986. A significant finding was that the hospital fact sheet, which is used to supply statistics to the CDC, understated the percentages of circumcisions done. The investigators had reviewed the total record to arrive at the circumcision rates of 89% and 84%, but had they only looked at the diagnosis on the discharge sheet, the rate would only have been about 70%; in 16% of the time the circumcision was recorded in the chart but not transcribed to the sheet used to determine statistics. This suggests that the true percentage of circumcisions done in the U.S. is higher than the figures cited by the CDC/NCHS, since these figures are only based on the data from the face sheet of the newborn record and not from the entire record. Supporting the high circumcision rates in Texas and Georgia are published data from Southern California which compared circumcision rates from a suburban practice, from a population consisting mainly of Hispanic babies and from a clinic serving mainly African Americans. In the suburban practice 83% chose circumcision, the circumcision rate was only 16% in the Hispanic group and 49% in the African Americans. Parental satisfaction was assessed in 68 families who left their sons uncircumcised and in 81 families who chose circumcision. When the boy was age 6-36 months the families who chose to leave their sons uncircumcised were significantly less satisfied with their decision than were the families electing circumcision. Confirming the high prevalence of circumcision in pediatric practices was a 1987 publication from Denver, Colorado which found that 80% of 124 infant boys were circumcised. As was noted above, this study found that the main factor in deciding was the circumcision status of the father. The pattern of high circumcision rates in non-Hispanic whites from pediatric practices was confirmed by evidence from San Francisco General Hospital, which has a lower socioeconomic clientele; in this population 76% of whites were circumcised as compared to 23% of Hispanics.

These reports provide firm evidence from governmental and clinical practice sources on the pattern and prevalence of circumcision in the U.S. Information from the CDC shows that about 65% of newborn boys nationwide are circumcised before they go home from the birthing hospital and this figure has remained unchanged for the past 2 decades. Clinical practice experience shows that in actuality about 80% of U.S males are circumcised. A 2005 poll of parents by American Baby magazine found that 82% had their newborn sons circumcised, a figure almost identical to the more scientific published studies in California, Texas, Colorado and Georgia which were cited above. The reasons for this discrepancy are clear. The CDC figures leave out boys who are circumcised after they leave the hospital. Jews and Moslems, who are circumcised later, are not counted, nor are other males who are circumcised for medical reasons or personal preference. Even in the case of newborn hospital circumcision, not all cases are included in data sent to the government, since, as was found in the Georgia study, circumcisions described in the record may not be transcribed to the sheet used for statistical purposes. A good example is the 92% circumcision rate in the Wisconsin community served by Dr. Robert Van Howe, a local pediatrician who is strongly opposed to circumcision: this makes sense in view of the 82% newborn hospital rate in the Midwest.

What is the outlook for the future of circumcision in the U.S.? I think the answer lies in the report from Denver, citing an 80% circumcision rate, which found that parents based their decision on social concerns rather than on medical ones. The circumcision status of the father was the main determining factor. The authors described the decision to circumcise as a cultural one in this country. This explains the continued high prevalence of circumcision in the U.S. despite strong opposition from highly organized activist anti-circumcision groups and the media, as well as the antipathy and disinterest of the American Academy of Pediatrics and other professional groups. Among non-immigrant groups the circumcision rate seems to be rising, as evidenced by increased circumcision in the Midwest and the South, which seems to offset or outweigh the fall in prevalence in States with high immigrant populations. It is interesting to note that even among Hispanics, who now comprise the largest number of births of any ethnic group in California, there are signs of increased interest in circumcision as they become "Americanized." Although the circumcision rate is essentially zero in Mexico, the native country of most California Hispanics, the rate was found to be 14% in the county hospital in Los Angeles and 23% at San Francisco General Hospital. I believe that as they spend more time in this country more Hispanics will adopt newborn circumcision, just as they do other aspects of our culture. After all, non-Hispanic whites in the Midwest have backgrounds from Europe where newborn circumcision was and is not performed, and almost all of them are now being circumcised. The predominance of circumcision in the U.S. has occurred in spite of the lack of awareness of the public and the profession of the multiple medical benefits of circumcision. Now that these lifetime medical benefits are increasingly being documented and the issue of pain has been addressed by local anesthesia, I think we will be seeing a further increase in the number of U.S. parents choosing to have newborn sons circumcised, and a greater interest in other countries around the world.

14

Religion, History and Culture

Since I am a pediatrician and not a religious figure, historian, or sociologist, I will cover history, religion, and culture only as they relate to the health aspects of modern day medical circumcision. Circumcision has been performed for thousands of years, and was practiced by the ancient Egyptians even before it became a religious ritual of Judaism, and later of Islam. Jews began to circumcise all male infants on the 8th day of life at the time of Abraham, as a covenant with God (Genesis, Chapter 17). As a Jew, Jesus was circumcised according to this ritual (Luke, Chapter 2 Verse 21), as were all the Apostles and early Christians. It wasn't until Paul (born Simon) was on his journey of proselytizing and conversion that it was decided that circumcision was not necessary to become a Christian. Paul wasn't born until 10 years after the death of Jesus, so for the first decades of Christianity all converts followed the rituals of Judaism, including circumcision, and essentially became Jews on their way to Christianity. This was the policy advocated by James, the brother of Jesus, and the early Church which was based in Jerusalem. Paul came back from his missionary journey of gaining converts in order to convince the Church in Jerusalem to drop circumcision as a requirement of Christianity. It has been stated that Paul was a "genius of practical evangelism," and he saw clearly that requiring circumcision would vastly impede the appeal of his gospel. The success of his mission, and those since, confirmed the wisdom of this decision in promoting the growth of Christianity. Jesus was born, lived and died as a Jew, but after circumcision was dropped at the behest of Paul, Christianity became more and more distanced from its Jewish roots. Circumcision is an integral part of Islam as well, and Mohammed was circumcised, although it is not clear whether he was born circumcised or was circumcised on the 7th day of life. Mohammed revered the prophet Abraham of the Old Testament as a guide and a model for the Muslim people, and circumcision is part of Islam. Muslims are circumcised but the various sects circumcise at different ages, from infancy to early adulthood.

In order to understand the origin of secular circumcision in the United States it is necessary to fast forward to the mid-nineteenth century and the medical practice and beliefs at the time. The current practice of circumcising almost all U.S. boys as a health measure began in the late 1800s as the result of the influence of some of America's most noted physicians. These included Drs. Lewis Sayre, J. Henry C. Simes, Norman H. Chapman, J. M. McGee and Peter Remondino, as well as a prominent British physician, Oliver H. Fowler. Some of the statements of these well known physicians seem remarkable and predictive in the light of current evidence over 100 years later. Sayre emphasized that circumcision was a prophylactic procedure against a wide variety of disorders. Performing surgery to prevent future disease was a new concept. Prevention of penile cancer and the problems of phimosis were 2 of the benefits cited. Simes is quoted as saying: "The operation of circumcision is one which may be performed for moral reasons; one which is demanded for hygienic purposes; one which is frequently necessary for pathological conditions; and, finally, one which is of unquestionably prophylactic importance." McGee favored the procedure as a sanitary precaution; "Circumcision, in a word, made the patient cleaner." Chapman regarded circumcision as a preventive, hygienic measure that would contribute to public health. Peter Remondino may have had the most influence in the U.S. since he presented his arguments in favor of circumcision in a book entitled *History of Circumcision from the Earliest Times to the Present: Moral and Physical Reasons for its Performance* which was first printed in 1891, and had a number of subsequent printings. Dr. Remondino, who lived in San Diego and was a Vice President of the California Medical Association, first presented his views to the Southern California Medical Association in 1889 in a talk entitled "A Plea for Circumcision; or the Dangers That Arise from the Prepuce." Not only did Remondino recognize the benefits of circumcision, but he described the mechanisms by which circumcision exerted its benefits. In cancer of the penis he proposed chronic infection as the cause, although he thought that herpes was the offending agent (human papilloma virus wasn't known)—"repeated attacks of herpes preputialis and some consequent point of induration are looked upon as starting points for the cancerous affection of the penis." As for syphilis, Remondino stated that "The retention of the virus (syphilis) is seemingly assisted by the topographical condition of the prepuce and its absorption is facilitated by the thinness of the mucous membrane. The absence of the prepuce and the non-absorbing character of the skin of the glans causes less tendency to favor syphilitic inoculation." Well stated and right on! I don't think we could describe it any more accurately today for any of the STDs that enter through the thin, often abraded foreskin membrane. In his Presidential Address to the Gloucester Branch of the British Medical Association in 1895 Dr. Oliver Fowler recommended universal prophylactic circumcision for reason of cleanliness. He stated that: "No one who has seen the superior cleanliness of a Hebrew penis can have avoided a very strong impression in favour of the removal of the foreskin. It constitutes a harbour for filth and is a constant source of irritation. It increases the risk of syphilis in early life and cancer in the aged. I have never seen cancer of the penis in a Jew, and chancres are rare."

The prominence of these physicians and the forcefulness of the message, particularly the dual advantages of health and hygiene, resonated on the middle class population of the time. It was an era of cleanliness being next to Godliness, and a procedure which could help keep the penis clean for a lifetime had a strong appeal. At this time during the turn of the century the popularity of newborn circumcision began among higher socioeconomic level families, and grew rapidly during the first half of the 20th century.

But the medical pioneers of circumcision were not perfect and they had some mistaken ideas as well. After all they were products of Victorian times. Policies were made on the basis of clinical experience and the biases of society, including moral judgments. Evidence-based medicine, clinical trials and outcome studies had not yet arrived. So, in addition to the predictive and clinically accurate observations on hygiene, phimosis, local infections, syphilis, and penile cancer, some of the distinguished physicians recommending routine newborn circumcision, particularly Sayre and Remondino, added some erroneous and baseless reasons for the procedure. These myths included the contention that the presence of the foreskin encouraged masturbation, which was looked upon as a dangerous condition which could lead to mental abnormalities. Further, it was claimed the "irritation" caused by the foreskin could lead to a large variety of neurological abnormalities from irritability to insanity and paralysis.

The present day opponents of circumcision argue that the reason why the American public began to choose newborn circumcision at the end of the 19th century, and from then on, was because they thought it would prevent masturbation and insanity. Although a few parents might have made the circumcision decision on the basis of preventing masturbation, subsequent evidence shows that the choice was made on the basis of health and hygiene by the overwhelming number of parents. As the 20th century progressed, and the myths of relationships between the foreskin and masturbation, insanity or neurological disorders were discredited, the prevalence of circumcision grew nevertheless. Better health and cleanliness were the predominant reasons for newborn circumcision given by the audience as they contradicted the anti-circumcision "experts" on the *Phil Donohue Show* in 1987 just as they were more than 100 years ago. If one looks at standard references pertaining to circumcision in the early part of the 20th century, health and cleanliness are emphasized, not masturbation. In the 1910-11 edition of the *Encyclopedia Britannica,* after going into the religious aspects of circumcision, it is stated that "as regards the non-ritual use of newborn circumcision, it may be added that in recent years the medical profession has been responsible for its considerable extension among other than Jewish children, the operation being recommended not merely in cases of malformation, but for reasons of health." In the 14th edition of the encyclopedia in 1929 it says "The operation is performed chiefly for purposes of cleanliness," and "In India the Hindus who do not circumcise ritually suffer far more frequently from cancer of the penis than the Mohammedans who circumcise." No mention of masturbation anywhere. Health and hygiene notwithstanding the main reason most parents choose circumcision for their sons is that they don't want the boys to look different from their fathers or from other boys. This could be termed the "locker room/father-son phenomenon."

One of the arguments that opponents of circumcision give

in the media to show that circumcision should be dropped in the U.S. is that "85% of the rest of the world doesn't circumcise." I don't think you are helping your cause with this statement, folks. The American public doesn't take well to the idea of using the rest of the world as a model. U.S parents don't want to follow the health practices of millions of "intact" Hindus in the ghettos of India, or of the hordes of uncircumcised peasants in China. We feel that the U.S. is the medical leader of the world, and rightly so. The rest of the world usually follows us, not the other way around. But what about Europe? Western European countries have excellent heath care systems, but newborn circumcision is almost never performed there. Here is where the "locker room phenomenon" comes in, in reverse. In the U.S. being circumcised means looking like your father, and the other boys and men, while conformity in Europe means having a foreskin. These situations tend to be self-perpetuating. If a U.S. boy is seen to be uncircumcised, the supposition is that he is an immigrant or the son of recent immigrants, not a position most young American boys are happy to embrace. The exception to the foreign origin revelation is in the case of sons of parents who have adopted the NOCIRC "intact" philosophy, a small group limited to certain enclaves on both coasts. On the basis of my clinical experience I can offer a profile of an uncircumcised non-immigrant American boy, not an uncommon sight in this Northern California area. Such a boy typically is the son of politically liberal, middle class, college educated parents with a common life style. They tend to be 'trendy" and live in certain coastal regions of the U.S. (particularly Berkeley, San Francisco, Marin County, the Los Angeles area (Hollywood, Beverly Hills), and the New York City suburbs such as Westchester County and Long Island). They are more likely to be vegetarians and peace activists and live in the "blue states." The highest circumcision rates are in the "red

states." Secular Jews are well represented among parents electing to leave their sons uncircumcised. Fashion and trends trump
tradition. I sometimes think that it is less likely that a male infant will be circumcised if his parents are secular Jews living
in Berkeley than if they are Conservative Christians in rural
Wisconsin. These "intact" groups, which have been successful
targets of the anti-circumcision groups are small in number,
and have had no significant impact on national circumcision
rates. This is indicated by the evidence that the circumcision
rate among non-immigrant American boys has not fallen, and
is actually rising slowly in spite of the growth and intense media
activities of the anti-circumcision groups.

In Europe the situation is very different. The rare circumcised boy has always been considered to be a Jew, a status
to which few European boys aspire, even in the absence of
anti-Semitism. In Nazi Germany an Aryan boy who required
a medical circumcision was presented with a major problem
in the locker room. The answer was that a non-Jewish male
who was circumcised during Hitler times was issued a certificate by the physician to show that he was not Jewish, and
listing the medical reason for circumcision. This was an important identity card to carry at all times, but I suspect that
even with this certificate a circumcised German boy of that
era would not be looked on with favor when applying to the
Hitler Youth or the SS. With the influx of Arab immigrants
into Western Europe in recent years, a circumcised boy in
the locker room today would more likely be a Muslim than a
Jew, but still would not be looked upon as a person to emu-
late by non-Muslim, non-Jewish European boys.

What about the contention that there is a Jewish influence in the U.S. which is responsible for the widespread use
of circumcision? There is no evidence to support this claim.
The contrary is more likely. Currently, Jewish physicians
have their greatest influence in the anti-circumcision move-

ment. Examples are Drs. Dean Edell, Paul Fleiss and Michael
Rothenberg (who has updated Dr. Spock's book with an anti-
circumcision twist). Two Jewish non-physicians, Ron Gold-
man and Edward Wallerstein have written anti-circumcision
books. It should be pointed out that 95% of circumcised
American boys are not Jewish (about 75% of U.S. males are
circumcised, but Jews make up only 3% of the population of
the country). Unlike in Europe being circumcised in the U.S.
is not a marker for being Muslim or Jewish. There were no
Jews among the group of influential physicians who were responsible for introducing circumcision to the U.S. in the 19th
century—Sayre, Simes, Chapman, McGee and Remondino.
The key 20th century physicians providing evidence on penile
cancer (Dean), HIV (Cameron and Plummer), cervical cancer (Castellsague) and infant kidney infection (Wiswell) were
all non-Jews. To digress briefly, an anti-circumcision article
alleged that there is a pro-circumcision conspiracy led by
"Jewish doctors, columnists, writers, politicians and clergy."
Those charged as part of this plot include "Dr. Aaron Fink,
Dear Abby, Ann Landers, Dr. June Reinisch, Dr. Julian Ansell, Dr. Tom Wiswell, Dr. Ruth and others." Since I am Jewish I don't know whether I should be grateful or disappointed
that I was not listed. On the other hand my friend Dr. Tom
Wiswell was surprised to find out that anti-circumcision activists had involuntarily converted him to Judaism. I have always considered that Tom, a West Point graduate and retired
Army doctor, was as good an example of a WASP (White
Anglo-Saxon Protestant) as one could find. Since a fair number of physicians are Jews, it is not surprising that they will
be represented among physicians favoring circumcision as
well as those opposed to the procedure. But why would a
Jewish physician try to impose circumcision on non-Jews? It
doesn't make sense. First of all Jews don't proselytize. How
many Jewish missionaries do you know? As a matter of fact

some potential converts to Judaism claim that it isn't easy—the Rabbis make it tough. Then it comes down to the selling points. Religions that are successful in gaining converts have very reassuring messages. Join my religion and find everlasting peace. Join my religion and go to heaven. Join my religion and be saved. But join my religion and get circumcised? I don't think so. As a matter of fact in the early days of Christianity Paul took the opposite tack with great success—you no longer have to get circumcised to join our religion. I doubt if preaching the virtues of circumcision will gain very many Jewish converts. So much for the Jewish connection or lack thereof.

What we're left with is the conclusion that in the U.S. newborn circumcision is well established, with a firm historical precedent, and is unrelated to religion. The presence of a foreskin in this country is most often a marker for an immigrant or the son of recent immigrants. Circumcision has become part of the American way of life and it is likely to not only remain so but to become even more popular as the evidence of multiple medical benefits continues to mount.

15

Summing Up:
What Was, What Is and What Will Be

In Part 1 of the book ("Proof") I presented objective scientific evidence and research studies relating the foreskin to a wide variety of disorders. Part 2 ("Consequences") was devoted to other factors that determine the acceptance of circumcision by the public. Politics, religion, history, social trends, and media coverage all play a role.

Only in America. The U.S. is the sole country in the world where secular circumcision is the policy of choice for the great majority of males. Most of the circumcisions here occur in the newborn period, but at least 10% are performed in older infants, children or adults. Outside the U.S. circumcision is done largely for religious or cultural reasons at various times of life (from the newborn period in Jews to various ages later in childhood for Muslims and certain cultural groups). The special position of circumcision in the U.S. results from a combination of medical evidence and social factors which are unique in this land of freedom and independence—openness to new ideas, willingness to change, tolerance, and self determination.

The pioneering physicians who first advocated secular circumcision(Simes, Chapman, McGee, Sayre, and Remondino), beginning in the middle of the 19th century, were among the most prominent in this country and highly respected by their colleagues and the public. Their recommendations were made on the premise that circumcision results in improved health and cleanliness. Their opinions on the benefits of circumcision were not based on scientific studies but rather on astute clinical observations, but they had it right. They recognized that circumcision was important in the prevention of phimosis, foreskin infections, syphilis and penile and cervical cancer. Clinical research and other objective studies over more than 100 years have proven them correct. On the other hand, they were wrong in claiming that circumcision prevented masturbation and emotional and neurological disorders. But it must be remembered that they lived in a different era and these erroneous impressions were not the reasons why middle class parents chose circumcision in increasing numbers. Better health and hygiene were and are the reasons given by the general public for choosing newborn circumcision in this country from the 19th century right up to the present.

By the early 1900's about 10% of non-Jewish males, mainly the offspring of educated middle class parents, were being circumcised in infancy and the trend has been upward ever since. By the end of World War II, in 1945, the great majority of American males were circumcised. Currently, if a male is uncircumcised in this country, it usually means he is either an immigrant, the son of recent immigrants, or his parents are among the small group of trendy "contrarians" in some communities who are influenced by the organized anti-circumcision groups. In Europe, on the other hand, a circumcised man is the exception, and in the past it generally meant he was a Jew (today he is more likely to be a Muslim), or a case where circumcision was performed as a medical necessity. Since most Americans are of European ancestry, how did this state of affairs come about? In Europe parents did not choose circumcision for their sons, but when they migrated to America they did. The answer, in my opinion, reflects the openness, willingness to change, lack of bias and acceptance of a new freedom and life style that has always characterized immigrants to this land. The limitations of class distinction and old world habits were left behind. Never mind that circumcision previously was performed only as a religious or cultural rite. Here it was thought to promote cleanliness and health, was recommended by leading U.S. physicians, and was the choice of well-to-do parents for their newborn boys. It was the thing to do in America. Circumcised sons of uncircumcised fathers were evidence of adaptation to a new land and a new style of life. As the procedure caught on it became self-perpetuating. If you left your sons uncircumcised you were clinging to the Old World ways.

The validity of this lifestyle change has been reinforced by a steadily increasing body of clinical research and scientific evidence confirming the multiple lifetime benefits of newborn circumcision. These range from prevention of urinary tract infections and local foreskin infections in infants and children, to penile cancer in old age, and sexually transmitted diseases (particularly HIV infection) in between. In the early 20th century important evidence was found in a national survey of cancer of the penis which showed that all cases in the U.S. occurred in uncircumcised men. This was confirmed by many other studies, every one of which showed that this devastating genital cancer was almost totally preventable by circumcision. An important discovery was that both penile cancer and uterine cervical cancer are caused by the same virus, human papilloma virus (HPV), and HPV is more commonly found on the penis of an uncircumcised man. Having an uncircumcised man as a sexual partner places a woman at increased risk for cervical cancer. In the early days of World War II, during the North African campaign in the desert, the loss of soldiers from combat due to foreskin infections resulted in the decision to circumcise many recruits at stateside training centers prior to being sent overseas. Military surgeons also found evidence to indicate that uncircumcised men were more likely to contract certain sexually transmitted diseases, particularly syphilis and chancroid, in which tearing of the delicate inner lining of the foreskin allowed the infection to enter. Pediatricians became most interested in circumcision by the discovery in the 1980's that severe kidney infections during the first year of life were about 10 times as common in uncircumcised infants. These infections developed after dangerous bacteria were found to bind to the moist inner surface of the foreskin but not to the circumcised penis. Unlike mild urinary infections later in childhood, which are more common in girls and do not seem to lead to long term damage, these male infant infections were found to frequently result in evidence of renal scarring, with the possibility of kidney failure later in life. The finding with the greatest potential benefit of circumcision to mankind was the observation in 1987 in sub-Saharan Africa that uncircumcised men were more likely to acquire HIV infection after sexual exposure than were circumcised men. Over 40 separate studies since then, extending to the present time, have found that uncircumcised men are 2-7 times at greater risk. Universal circumcision could save millions of lives in Africa and Asia. Scientific studies have shown that HIV enters the body by binding to specialized cells in the foreskin. As is the case with bacteria in infant urinary infections, the foreskin acts as a magnet for the virus in HIV. These are the proven preventive health advantages of newborn circumcision. They are documented in Part I and in the Reference section.

What has been the response of the medical profession to this overwhelming evidence of multiple preventive health benefits of newborn circumcision, benefits which begin in early infancy and extend through the lifetime of the boy? Not what it should be. Modern day physicians from the 1970s to the present have had less insight and interest in the medical importance of circumcision than did their contemporaries in the late 19th century, and less than the general public for that matter. I think the reason is the rapid growth of medical sub-specialization—what has been referred to as knowing more and more about less and less. There are now few physicians who look at the total picture unlike the professional giants of 100 years ago, upon whose shoulders they stand. American pediatricians may know about infant urinary tract infections (UTIs), but they have no knowledge or interest in penile and cervical cancer, let alone AIDS in Africa. They then conclude that circumcision does indeed prevent infant UTIs, but this is not sufficient reason to recommend the procedure. On the other hand geriatricians know that elderly circumcised men are protected from penile cancer, but are likely unaware and uninterested in the relationship between circumcision and infant UTIs, cervical cancer or HIV in young adults in Africa. Each specialty is isolated and territorial. And none more so than neotatologists, the hospital-based specialists charged with caring for immature and sick newborns. These experts on desperately ill babies are extremely dedicated pro-fessionals and have worked wonders on saving baby's lives. But they have less interest in normal newborns, and do not see them after they leave the hospital. Thus, they have no experience with any preventive health benefits of circumci-sion in infants, children or adults. On the other hand, since circumcisions are done in the nursery prior to discharge, they would see any ill effects or complications. Their professional territory permits them to observe all the bad effects of the procedure and none of the good. It is no wonder that neo-natologists have always been opposed to circumcision. What is unexplainable is how and why this highly biased group of professionals was the very one assigned the task of evaluat-ing and making recommendations for or against newborn circumcision. Therein lays the tale of the confusing and erroneous policies and statements of the American Academy of Pediatrics (AAP), detailed in Chapter 12.

The American public and the pioneering physicians of the 19th century took a simpler and broader view. They looked at the big picture. Each of the health benefits of circumcision wasn't considered alone. All the benefits were added together, and the sum led to the conclusion that a circumcised male was cleaner and healthier. The cleanliness issue was obvious 150 years ago just as it is today—it's easier to keep the penis clean if there is no foreskin to accumulate smegma and germs. During the years 1850-1900, clinical observation indicated that healthier meant prevention of phimosis, foreskin infections, penile cancer and probably cervical cancer and syphilis. One hundred years later, in 1999, the time of the most recent AAP report, clinical studies proved the value of these benefits. At least 2 new benefits were added, prevention of infant kidney infections and HIV. By 2004 there was further published proof regarding cervical cancer, penile cancer, HIV, and prevention of penile skin disorders. In addition, for the first time there were multiple objective studies in men circumcised as adults which showed no difference in sexual satisfaction with or without a foreskin, and women preferred the circumcised penis for esthetic reasons leading to more varied sex in circumcised men. The issue of pain was addressed by local anesthetic techniques, making painless newborn circumcision the standard of care. Today the American public may not be aware of all this evidence indicating more advantages of newborn circumcision than was known in the 19th century, but their conclusion is the same. Circumcision is cleaner and healthier now just as it was 150 years ago. The bottom line is that in the face of a strong lay anti-circumcision movement which dominates the media and the Internet, and a disinterested medical profession, more than 75% of U.S.

males are circumcised. This number is over 90% in some communities in Middle America.

How beneficial is circumcision in the United States? As a result of the predominance of circumcised males in this country infant boys under the age of 1 year are 10 times less likely to get severe kidney infections as their uncircumcised counterparts, young men are half as likely to acquire HIV infection when sexually exposed, women have twice the chance of avoiding cervical cancer, and older men are almost completely protected against cancer of the penis. As visible advantages of circumcision these values translate into annual figures of about 18,000 fewer cases of infant kidney infections, and avoidance of 15,000 HIV infections in men (with 3500 deaths), 6500 cervical cancers (with 2200 deaths) and 1200 penile cancers (with 200 deaths). And American circumcised men have cleaner penises, fewer local infections and rashes, and more varied sex.

It seems likely that as published proof on the substantial lifetime health benefits of newborn circumcision continues to accumulate, professional and public awareness will increase and the circumcision rate will go up even further, just as it has over the past 20 years in the Midwest and the South. As has been the case with European immigrants in the past, current Hispanic and Asian immigrants will probably have their sons circumcised as they remain in this country longer. This has already been happening with Hispanic immigrants who have a higher circumcision rate in Northern California (29% in San Francisco vs. essentially zero in the Southern California towns bordering Mexico). The new immigrants will accept that circumcision in this country is looked upon as a visible part of Americanization.

The saga of how an operative procedure, previously a religious and cultural rite, became a part of the culture of the U.S. over a period of more than 100 years is unique. It is a measure of the adaptability, common sense and willingness to change that characterize the citizens of this country. The story is one that is ongoing and could only happen here. It's as American as baseball, the stars and stripes, apple pie— and circumcision.

References

This Reference section is for those readers who would like to check the original publications and data referred to in the book. The References are organized to document each chapter, and are available in medical libraries, and in some cases online.

Chapter 1: Why Newborns? The Window of Opportunity.
1. Moore KL, Persaud TV. The developing human: clinically oriented embryology. 6th ed. Philadelphia: WB Saunders, 1998.
2. Brooks JD. Anatomy of the lower urinary tract and male genitalia. In: Walsh PC, Retik AB, Vaugh Jr, ED Wein AJ, eds. Campbell's Urology. 7th ed. Philadelphia: Saunders WB, 1998, pp 89-128.
3. Maizels M. Normal and anomalous development of the urinary tract. In: PC Walsh, Retik AB, Vaugh Jr ED, Wein AJ, eds. Campbell's Urology. 7th ed. Philadelphia: Saunders WB, 1998, pp 1545-1600.
4. Tanagho EA. Anatomy of the genitourinary tract. In: Tanagho EA, McAninch JW, eds. Smith's General Urology. 15th ed. New York: Lange Medical Books/McGraw-Hill, 2000, pp 1-16.
5. Tanagho EA. Embrology of the genitourinary system. In: Tanagho EA, McAninch JW, eds. Smith's General Urology. 15th ed. New York: Lange Medical Books/McGraw-Hill, 2000, pp 17-30.
6. Altemus AR, Hutchins GM. Development of the human anterior urethra. J Urol 146:1085-1093, 1991.
7. Blass EM, Hoffmeyer LB. Sucrose as an analgesic for newborn infants. Pediatrics 87:215-218, 1991.

Chapter 2: What Is Circumcision? Why Do It? How To Do It, and What Can Go Wrong?
1. Kurtis PS, DeSilva HN, Bernstein BA, Malakh L, Schechter NL. A comparison of Mogen and Gomco clamps in combination with dorsal penile

nerve block in minimizing the pain of neonatal circumcision. Pediatrics 103:E23.

2. Gee WF, Ansell JS. Neonatal circumcision: a ten-year overview: with comparison of the Gomco clamp and the Plastibell device. Pediatrics 58:824-827, 1976.

3. Stang HJ, Snellman LW, Condon LM, Conroy MM, Liebo R, Brodersen L, Gunnar MR. Beyond dorsal penile nerve block: a more humane circumcision. Pediatrics 100:E3, 1997.

4. Fontaine P, Toffler WL. Dorsal penile nerve block for newborn circumcision. Am Fam Physician 43:1327-1333, 1991.

5. Taddio A, Pollock N, Gilbert-Macleod C, Ohlsson K, Koren G. Combined analgesia and local anesthesia to minimize pain during circumcision. Arch Pediatr Adolesc Med 154:620-623, 2000.

6. Blass EM, Hoffmeyer LB. Sucrose as an analgesic for newborn infants. Pediatrics 87:215-218, 1991.

7. Butler-O'Hara M, LeMoine C, Guillet R.. Analgesia for neonatal circumcision: a randomized controlled trial of EMLA cream versus dorsal penile nerve block.Pediatrics. 1998 Apr;101(4):E5.

8. al-Samarrai AY, Mofti AB, Crankson SJ, Jawad A, Haque K, al-Meshari A. A review of a Plastibell device in neonatal circumcision in 2,000 instances. Surg Gynecol Obstet 1988; 167: 341-343.

9. Howard CR, Howard FM, Fortune K, Generalli P, Zolnoun D, ten Hoopen C, de Blieck E. A randomized, controlled trial of a eutectic mixture of local anesthetic cream (lidocaine and prilocaine) versus penile nerve block for pain relief during circircumcision. Am J Obstet Gynecol 1999; 181: 1506-1511.

10. Lander J, Metcalfe JB, Muttitt S, Brady-Fryer B. Local anaesthesia for infants undergoing circumcision. J Am Med Assoc 1998; 279: 1171.

Chapter 3: Infant Kidney Infections.

1. Wiswell TE, Miller GM, Gelston Jr HM, Jones SK, Clemmings AF. Effect of circumcision status on periurethral bacterial flora during the first year of life. J Pediatrc 113:442-446, 1988.

2. Wiswell TE. John K. Lattimer lecture. Prepuce presence portends prevalence of potentially perilous periurethral pathogens. J Urol 148:739-742, 1992.

3. Roberts JA. Does circumcision prevent urinary tract infection. J Urol 135:991-992, 1986.

4. Fussell EN, Kaack MB, Cherry R, Roberts JA. Adherence of bacteria to human foreskins. J Urol 140:997-1001, 1988.

5. Spach DH, Stapleton AE, Stamm WE. Lack of circumcision increases the risk of urinary tract infection in young men. JAMA 267:679-681, 1992.

6. Shaw KN, Gorelick M, McGowan KL, Yakscoe NM, Schwartz JS. Prevalence of urinary tract infection in febrile young children in the

emergency department. Pediatrics 102:E16, 1998.

7. Schoen EJ, Colby CJ, Ray GT. Newborn circumcision decreases incidence and costs of urinary tract infections during the first year of life. Pediatrics 105:789-793, 2000.

8. Jakobsson B, Esbjorner E, Hansson S. Minimum incidence and diagnostic rate of first urinary tract infection. Pediatrics 104:222-226, 1999.

9. Rushton HG, Majd M, Jantausch B, Wiedermann BL, Belman AB. Renal scarring following reflux and nonreflux pyelonephritis in children: evaluation with 99mtechnetium-dimercaptosuccinic acid scintigraphy [published erratum appears in J Urol, 148:898, 1992]. J Urol 47:1327-1332, 1992.

10. Stokland E, Hellstrom M, Jacobsson B, Jodal U, Sixt R. Renal damage one year after first urinary tract infection: role of dimercaptosuccinic acid scintigraphy. J Pediatr 129:815-820, 1996.

11. Rodriguez-Soriano J, Vallo A, Quintela MJ, Oliveros R, Ubetagoyena M. Normokalaemic pseudohypoaldosteronism is present in children with acute pyelonephritis. Acta Paediatr 81:402-406, 1992.

12. Schoen EJ, Bhatia S, Ray GT, Clapp W, To TT. Transient pseudohypoaldosteronism with hyponatremia-hyperkalemia in infant urinary tract infection. J Urol 167:680-682, 2002.

13. Craig JC, Knight JF, Sureshkumar P, Mantz E, Roy LP. Effect of circumcision on incidence of urinary tract infection in preschool boys. J Pediat 1996; 128: 23-27.

14. To T, Agha M, Dick PT, Feldman W. Cohort study on circumcision of newborn boys and subsequent risk of urinary tract infection. Lancet 1998; 352: 1113-1116.

15. Wiswell TE. The prepuce, urinary tract infections, and the consequences. Pediatrics 2000; 105: 8602.

16. Newman TB, Bernzweig JA, Takayama JI, Finch SA, Wasserman RC, Pantell RH. Urine testing and urinary tract infections in febrile infants seen in office settings: the Pediatric Research in Office Settings' Febrile Infant Study.

17. Hoberman A, Charron M, Hickey RW, Baskin M, Kearney DH, Wald ER. Imaging studies after a first febrile urinary tract infection in young children. N Engl J Med. 2003 Jan 16;348(3):195-202.

18. Patzer L, Seeman T, Luck C, Wuhl E, Janda J, Misselwitz J. Day- and night-time blood pressure elevation in children with higher grades of renal scarring. J Pediatr. 2003 Feb;142(2):117-22.

19. Schoen EJ. Benefits of newborn circumcision: is Europe ignoring medical evidence? Arch Dis Child. 1997 Sep;77(3):258-60.

Chapter 4: Local Penile Problems.

1. Kalcev B. Circumcision and personal hygiene in school boys. Med Officer 112:171-173, 1964.

2. Oster J. Further fate of the foreskin: incidence of preputial adhesions,

phimosis, and smegma among Danish school-boys. Arch Dis Child 43:200-203, 1968.

3. Escala JM, Rickwood AM. Balanitis. Br J Urol 63:196-197, 1989.

4. Frank R. Circumcision and hygiene in geriatric patients [letter]. J Am Geriatr Soc 47:1155, 1999.

5. Mallon E, Hawkins D, Dinneen M, Francics N, Fearfield L, Newson R, C Bunker. Circumcision and genital dermatoses. Arch Dermatol 136:350-354, 2000.

6. Shearn MA, Shearn L. Profile: Louis XVI. Medical Aspects of Human Sexuality 17:139-140, 1983.

7. English JC, Laws RA, Keough GC, Wilde JL, Foley JP, Elston DM. Dermatoses of the glans penis and prepuce. J Am Acad Dermatol 1997; 37: 1-24.

8. Fakjian N, Hunter S, Cole GW, Miller J. An argument for circumcision. Prevention of balanitis in the adult. Arch Dermatol 1990; 126: 1046-1047.

9. Gardner AMN. Circumcision and sand. J Roy Soc Med 1991; 84: 387.

10. Gunsar C, Kurutepe S, Alparslan O, Yulmaz O, Daglar Z, Sencan A, Genc A, Taneli C, Mir E. The effect of circumcision status on periurethral and glanular bacterial flora. Urol Int 2004; 72: 212-215.

11. Herzog LW, Alvarez SR. The frequency of foreskin problems in uncircumcised children. Am J Dis Child 1986; 140: 254-256.

12. Kohn F-M, Pflieger-Bruss S, Schill W-B. Penile skin diseases. Andrologia 1999; 31(suppl1): 3-11.

13. Winberg J, Bollgren I, Gothefors L, Herthelius M, Tullus K.The prepuce: a mistake of nature? Lancet. 1989 Mar 18;1(8638):598-9.

14. Shankar KR, Rickwood AM. The incidence of phimosis in boys. BJU Int. 1999 Jul;84(1):101-2.

15. Ridley CM. Genital lichen sclerosus (lichen sclerosus et atrophicus) in childhood and adolescence. J R Soc Med. 1993 Feb;86(2):69-75.

16. Kyriazi NC, Costenbader CL. Group A Group A beta-hemolytic streptococcal balanitis: it may be more common than you think. Pediatrics. 1991 Jul;88(1):154-6. Spilsbury K, Semmens JB, Wisniewski ZS, Holman CD. Circumcision for phimosis and other medical indications in Western Australian boys. Med J Aust. 2003 Feb 17;178(4):155-8.

Chapter 5: An Ignored Weapon Against HIV/AIDS.

1. Simonsen JN, Cameron DW, Gakinya MN, Ndinya-Achola JO, D'Costa LJ, Karasira P, Cheang M, Ronald AR, Piot P, Plummer FA. Human immunodeficiency virus infection among men with seuxally transmitted diseases. Experience from a center in Africa. N Engl J Med 319:274-278, 1988.

2. Cameron DW, Simonsen JN, D'Costa LJ, Ronald AR, Maitha GM, Gakinya MN, Cheang M, Ndinya-Achola JO, Piot P, Brunham RC, et

al. Female to male transmission of human immunodeficiency virus type 1: risk factors for seroconversion in men. Lancet 2:403-407, 1989.

3. Caldwell JC, Caldwell P. The African AIDS epidemic. Sci Am 274:62-63, 66-68, 1996.

4. Moses S, Plummer FA, Bradley JE, Ndinya-Achola JO, Nagelkerke NJ, Ronald AR. The association between lack of male circumcision and risk for HIV infection: a review of the epidemiological data. Sex Transm Dis 21:201-210, 1994.

5. Halperin DT, Bailey RC. Male circumcision and HIV infection: 10 years and counting. Lancet 354:1813-1815, 1999.

6. Potts M. Male circumcision and HIV infection [letter]. Lancet 355:926-7, discussion 927, 2000.

7. Kreiss JK, Hopkins SG. The association between circumcision status and human immunodeficiency virus infection among homosexual men. J Infect Dis 168:1404-1408, 1993.

8. Bailey RC. Male circumcision as an effective HIV prevention strategy: Current evidence. 8th Conference on Retroviruses and Opportunistic Infections, Chicago 2001; S22: http://www.retroconference.org//requested_lectures.cfm?ID=383& mode =send.

9. Bailey RC, Muga R, Poulussen R, Abicht H. The acceptability of male circumcision to reduce HIV infections in Nyanza Province, Kenya. AIDS Care 2002; 14: 27-40.

10. Szabo R, Short RV. How does male circumcision protect against HIV infection? BMJ 320:1592-1594, 2000.

11. Patterson BK, Landay A, Siegel JN, Flener Z, Pessis D, Chaviano A, Bailey RC. Susceptibility to human immunodeficiency virus-1 infection of human foreskin and cervical tissue grown in explant culture. Am J Pathol 161:867-873, 2002.

12. Drain PK, Smith JS, Hughes JP, Halperin DT, Holmes KK. Correlates of national HIV seroprevalence: An ecologic analysis of 122 developing countries. J Acquir Immune Defic Syndr 2004; 35: 407-420.

13. Kebaabetswe P, Lockman S, Mogwe S, Mandevu R, Thior I, Essex M, Shapiro RL. Male circumcision: an acceptable strategy for HIV prevention in Botswana. Sex Transm Infect 2003; 79: 214-219.

14. Lagarde E, Dirk T, Puren A, Reathe RT, Bertran A. Acceptability of male circumcision as a tool for preventing HIV infection in a highly infected community in South Africa. AIDS 2003; 17: 89-95.

15. Rain-Taljaard RC, Lagarde E, Taljaard DJ, Campbell C, MacPhail C, Williams B, Auvert B. Potential for an intervention based on male circumcision in a South African town with high levels of HIV infection. AIDS Care 2003; 15: 315-327.

16. Short RV. The HIV/AIDS pandemic: New ways of preventing infection in men. Reprod Fert Devel 2004; 16: 555-559.

17. Hyena H. Is there a connection between AIDS and circumcision? Researchers claim decade-old evidence has been ignored. Salon.com,

Health & Body. Feb. 28,2000.

18. Halperin DT, Weiss HA, Hayes R, Auvert B, Bailey RC, Caldwell J, Coates T, Padian N, Potts M, Ronald A, Short R, Williams B, Klausner J. Response to Ronald Gray, Male circumcision and HIV acquisition and transmission: cohort studies in Rakai, Uganda (2000, 14:2371-2381). AIDS. 2002 Mar 29;16(5):810-2; author reply 809-10.

19. Gray RH, Kiwanuka N, Quinn TC, Sewankambo NK, Serwadda D, Mangen FW, Lutalo T, Nalugoda F, Kelly R, Meehan M, Chen MZ, Li C, Wawer MJ. Male circumcision and HIV acquisition and transmission: cohort studies in Rakai, Uganda. Rakai Project Team. AIDS. 2000 Oct 20;14(15):2371-81.

20. Halperin DT, Epstein H. Concurrent sexual partnerships help to explain Africa's high HIV prevalence: implications for prevention. Lancet. 2004 Jul 3;364(9428):4-6.

21. Halperin DT, Post GL. Global HIV prevalence: the good news might be even better. Lancet. 2004 Sep 18;364(9439):1035-6.

22. Stephenson J. New HIV prevention strategies urged: averting new infections key to controlling pandemic. JAMA. 2004 Sep 8;292(10):1163-4.

23. Agot KE, Ndinya-Achola JO, Kreiss JK, Weiss NS. Risk of HIV-1 in rural Kenya: a comparison of circumcised and uncircumcised men. Epidemiology. 2004 Mar;15(2):157-63.

24. Halperin DT. Male Circumcision and HIV Prevention. Washington, DC; USAID Bureau of Global Health (August 2003). http://www.rho.org/html/menrh_mtg_mc_09_02.html#usaid03

Chapter 6: Other Sexually Transmitted Diseases (STDs).

1. Wilson RA. Circumcision and venereal disease. Can Med Assoc J 56:54-56, 1947.

2. Taylor PK, Rodin P. Herpes genitalis and circumcision. Br J Vener Dis 51:274-277, 1975.

3. Parker SW, Stewart AJ, Wren MN, Gollow MM, Straton JA. Circumcision and sexually transmissible disease. Med J Aust 2:288-290, 1983.

4. Basset I, Donovan B, Bodsworth NJ, Field PR, Ho DW, Jeansson S, Cunningham AL. Herpes simplex virus type 2 infection of heterosexual men attending a sexual health centre. Med J Aust 1994; 160: 697-700.

5. Cook LS, Koutsky LA, Homes KK. Circumcision and sexually transmitted diseases. Am J Public Health 84:197-201, 1994.

6. Moses S, Bailey RC, Ronald AR. Male circumcision: assessment of health risks and benefits. Sex Transm Infect 74:368-373, 1998.

7. Diseker RA, Peterman TA, Kamb ML, Kent C, Zenilman JM, Douglas JM, Rhodes F, Iatesta M. Circumcision and STD in the United States: Cross sectional and cohort analysis. Sex Transm Infect 2000; 76: 474-479.

8. Cherpes TL, Meyn LA, Krohn MA, Hillier SL. Risk factors for infection

with herpes simplex virus type 2: role of smoking, douching, uncircumcised males, and vaginal flora. Sex Transm Dis. 2003 May;30(5):405-10.

9. Cook LS, Koutsky LA, Holmes KK. Circumcision and sexually transmitted diseases. Am J Public Health. 1994 Feb;84(2):197-201.

Chapter 7: Cancer of the Penis

1. Dean Jr AL. Epithelioma of the penis. J Urol 33:252-283, 1935.

2. Plaut A, Kohn-Speyer AC. The carcinogenic action of smegma. Science 105:391-392, 1947.

3. Dagher R, Selzer ML, Lapides J. Carcinoma of the penis and the anticircumcision crusade. J Urol 110:79-80, 1973.

4. Kochen M, McCurdy S. Circumcision and the risk of cancer of the penis: a life-table analysis. Am J Dis Child 134:484-486, 1980.

5. Leiter E, Lefkovits AM. Circumcision and penile carcinoma. NY State J Med 75:1520-1522, 1975.

6. Schoen EJ. The relationship between circumcision and cancer of the penis. CA Cancer J Clin 41:306-309, 1991.

7. Schoen EJ, Oehrli M, Colby CJ, Machin G. The highly protective effect of newborn circumcision against invasive penile cancer. Pediatrics 105: E36, 2000.

8. Gajalakshmi CK, Shanta V. Association between cervical and penile cancers in Madras, India. Acta Oncologica 32:617-620, 1993.

9. American Cancer Society. Cancer statistics. 2004; http://www.cancer.org/docroot/CRI/content/CRI_2_4_1X_What_are_the_key_statistics_for_penile_cancer_35.asp?sitearea=.

10. Boon ME, Susanti I, Tasche MJ, Kok LP. Human papillomavirus (HPV) associated male and female genital carcinomas in a Hindu population. The male as a vector and victim. Cancer 1989; 64: 550-565.

11. Gross G, Pfister H. Role of human papillomavirus in penile cancer, penile intraepithelial squamous cell neoplasias and in genital warts. Med Microbiol Immunol 2004; 193: 35-44.

12. McCance DJ, Kalache A, Ashdown K, Andrade L, Menezes F, Smith P, Doll R. Human papillomavirus types 16 and 18 in carcinoma of the penis from Brazil. J Cancer 1986; 37: 55-59.

13. Pratt-Thomas HR, Heins HC, Latham E, Dennis EJ, McIver FA. Carcinogenic effect of human smegma: An experimental study. Cancer 1956; 9: 671-680.

14. Reddy DG, Baruah IK. Carcinogenic action of human smegma. Arch Pathol 1963; 75: 414.

15. Villa LL, Lopez A. Human papillomavirus sequence in penile carcinomas in Brazil. Int J Cancer 1986; 37: 853-855.

16. World Health Organization, International Agency for Research on Cancer. Cancer Incidence in Five Countries. International Agency for Research on Cancer. Vol. vol 1 – vol 7. 1966-1997.

17. Brinton LA, Li JY, Rong SD, Huang S, Xiao BS, Shi BG, Zhu ZJ, Schiffman MH, Dawsey S. Risk factors for penile cancer: results from a case-control study in China. Int J Cancer. 1991 Feb 20;47(4):504-9.

18. Cupp MR, Malek RS, Goellner JR, Smith TF, Espy MJ.The detection of human papillomavirus deoxyribonucleic acid in intraepithelial, in situ, verrucous and invasive carcinoma of the penis.J Urol. 1995 Sep;154(3):1024-9. Review.

19. Hardner GJ, Bhanalaph T, Murphy GP, Albert DJ, Moore RH. Carcinoma of the penis: analysis of therapy in 100 consecutive cases. J Urol. 1972 Sep;108(3):428-30. No abstract available.

20. Malek RS, Goellner JR, Smith TF, Espy MJ, Cupp MR. Human papillomavirus infection and intraepithelial, in situ, and invasive carcinoma of penis. Urology. 1993 Aug;42(2):159-70. Review. Erratum in: Urology 1994 Jan;43(1):followi.

21. Holly EA, Palefsky JM. Factors related to risk of penile cancer: new evidence from a study in the Pacific Northwest. J Natl Cancer Inst. 1993 Jan 6;85(1):2-4.

22. Persky L, deKernion J. Carcinoma of the penis. CA Cancer J Clin. 1986 Sep-Oct;36(5):258-73.

23. Sanders CJ. Condylomata acuminata of the penis progressing rapidly to invasive squamous cell carcinoma. Genitourin Med. 1997 Oct;73(5):402-3.

24. Castellsagué X, Bosch FX, Muños N, Meijer CJ, Shah KV, de SanJosé S, Eluf-Neto J, Ngelangel CA, Chichareon S, Smith JS, et al. Male circumcision, penile human papillomavirus infection, and cervical cancer in female partners. N Engl J Med 346:1105-1112, 2002.

Chapter 8: Cancer of the Cervix in Female Partners.

1. Gajalakshmi CK, Shanta V. Association between cervical and penile cancers in Madras, India. Acta Oncologica 32:617-620, 1993.

2. Castellsagué X, Bosch FX, Muños N, Meijer CJ, Shah KV, de SanJosé S, Eluf-Neto J, Ngelangel CA, Chichareon S, Smith JS, et al. Male circumcision, penile human papillomavirus infection, and cervical cancer in female partners. N Engl J Med 346:1105-1112, 2002.

3. Adami HO, Trichopoulos D. Cervical cancer and the elusive male factor. N Engl J Med 146:1160-1161, 2002.

4. Cannistra SA, Niloff JM. Cancer of the uterine cervix. N Engl J Med. 1996 Apr 18;334(16):1030-8.

5. American Cancer Society. Cancer statistics. 2004; http://www.cancer.org/docroot/CRI/content/CRI_2_4_1X_What_are_the_key_statistics_for_penile_cancer_35.asp?sitearea=.

6. Boon ME, Susanti I, Tasche MJ, Kok LP. Human papillomavirus (HPV) associated male and female genital carcinomas in a Hindu population. The male as a vector and victim. Cancer 1989; 64: 550-565.

7. Walboomers JM, Jacobs MV, Manos MM, Bosch FX, Kummer JA,

Shah KV, Snijders PJ, Peto J, Meijer CJ, Munoz N. Human papilloma-virus is a necessary cause of invasive cervical cancer. J Pathol 1999; 189: 12-19.

8. World Health Organization, International Agency for Research on Can-cer. Cancer Incidence in Five Countries. International Agency for Re-search on Cancer. Vol. vol 1 – vol 7. 1966-1997.

9. Sun XW, Kuhn L, Ellerbrock TV, Chiasson MA, Bush TJ, Wright TC Jr. Human papillomavirus infection in women infected with the human immunodeficiency virus. N Engl J Med. 1997 Nov 6;337(19):1343-9.

10. zur Hausen H. Genital papillomavirus infections. Prog Med Virol. 1985; 32:15-21.

11. Wright TC Jr, Schiffman M. Adding a test for human papillomavi-rus DNA to cervical-cancer screening. N Engl J Med. 2003 Feb 6;348(6):489-90.

Chapter 9: Sex and Sensitivity

1. Masters WH, Johnson VE. Human Sexual Response, Little, Brown and Company, Boston, 1966, p.190.

2. Williamson ML, Williamson PS. Women's preferences for penile cir-cumcision in sexual partners. J Sex Educ Ther 14:8-12, 1988.

3. Lue TF. Physiology of penile erection and pathophysiology of erectile dysfunction and priapism. In: PC Walsh, AB Retik, ED Vaugh Jr, AJ Wein, eds. Campbell's Urology. 7th ed. Philadelphia: WB Saunders, 1998, pp 1157-1180.

4. Collins S, Upshaw J, Rutchik S, Ohannessian C, Ortenberg J, Albertsen P. Effects of circumcision on male sexual function: debunking a myth? J Urol 167:2111-2112, 2002.

5. Fink KS, Carson CC, DeVellis RF. Adult circumcision outcomes study: effect on erectile function, penile sensitivity, sexual activity and satis-faction. J Urol 167:2113-2116, 2002.

6. Bluestein CB, Eckholdt H, Arezzo JC, Melman A. Effects of circum-cision on male penile sensitivity [abstract]. J Urol 169(4 Suppl):324, 2003.

7. Senkul T, Iseri C, Sen B, Karademir K, Saracoglu F, Erden D. Circumci-sion in adults: Effect on sexual function. Urology 2004; 63: 155-158.

8. Melman A. Improving Erectile Function: Detection, Prevention, and Treatment of ED. Amer Urological Association Meeting. April 2004

9. Laumann EO, Masi CM, Zuckerman EW. Circumcision in the United States. Prevalence, prophylactic effects, and sexual practice. JAMA 1997 Apr 2;277(13):1052-7.

10. Latif AS, Katzenstein DA, Bassett MT, Houston S, Emmanuel JC, Ma-rowa E. Genital ulcers and transmission of HIV among couples in Zim-babwe. AIDS 1989; 3: 519-523.

11. Laumann EO, Maal CM, Zuckerman EW. Circumcision in the United States. Prevalence, prophyactic effects, and sexual practice. J Am Med

Assoc 1997; 277: 1052-1057.

12. National Center for Health Statistics of the Department of Health and Human Services. Trends in Circumcisions Among Newborns. 2003; http://www.cdc.gov/nchs/products/pubs/pubd/hestats/circumcisions/ circumcisions.htm.

13. Vickers MA, Wright EA. Erectile dysfunction in the patient with diabetes mellitus. Am J Manag Care. 2004 Jan;10(1 Suppl):S3-11; quiz S12-6.

Chapter 10: Circumcision and the Military

1. Patton JF. Venereal disease. In: United States Army. Medical Dept. Surgery in World War II: Urology. Washington, DC: Office of the Surgeon General and Center of Military History, United States Army 1987, pp 45-88.

2. Stewart CM. Infections and related conditions. In: United States Army. Medical Dept. Surgery in World War II: Urology. Washington, DC: Office of the Surgeon General and Center of Military History, United States Army, 1987, pp 99-146.

3. Vermooten V. Genitourinary neoplasms. In: United States Army. Medical Dept. Surgery in World War II: Urology. Washington, DC: Office of the Surgeon General and Center of Military History, United States Army, 1987, pp 167-192.

4. Culp OS, Patton JF. Reflections. In: United States Army. Medical Dept. Surgery in World War II: Urology. Washington, DC: Office of the Surgeon General and Center of Military History, United States Army, 1987, pp 485-490.

Chapter 11: Non-Science, Nonsense, Quotes and Anecdotes
References in the text.

Chapter 12: American Academy of Pediatrics—Not It's Finest Hour

1. American Academy of Pediatrics. Committee on Fetus and Newborn. Standards and Recommendations for Hospital Care of Newborn Infants. 5th ed. Evanston, IL: American Academy of Pediatrics, 1971.

2. Thompson HC, King LR, Knox E, Korones SB. Report of the Ad Hoc Task Force on Circumcision. Pediatrics 56:610-611, 1975.

3. American Academy of Pediatrics: Report of the Task Force on Circumcision [Published erratum appears in Pediatrics, 84:761, 1989]. Pediatrics 84:388-391, 1989.

4. Circumcision policy statement. American Academy of Pediatrics. Task Force on Circumcision. Pediatrics 103:686-693, 1999.(American Academy of Pediatrics. Circumcision Information for Parents. Elk Grove Village: American Academy of Pediatrics, 1999).

5. Schoen EJ, Wiswell TE, Moses S. New policy on circumcision – Cause for concern. Pediatrics 2000; 105: 620-623.

6. Van Howe RS. Variability in penile appearance and penile findings: a prospective study. Br J Urol. 1997 Nov;80(5):776-82.
7. Brown MS, Brown CA. Circumcision decision: prominence of social concerns. Pediatrics. 1987 Aug;80(2):215-9.
8. Adler R, Ottaway MS, Gould S. Circumcision: we have heard from the experts; now let's hear from the parents.Pediatrics. 2001 Feb;107(2): E20.

Chapter 13: Circumcision Statistics: Don't Believe Everything You Hear
1. United States. National Center for Health Statistics. Trends in circumcisions among newborns [website]. Available from: URL: **http://www. cdc.gov/nchs/products/pubs/pubd/hestats/circumcisions/circumcisions.htm** (accessed November 11, 2001).
2. California. Department of Health Services. Vital Statistics Data Tables, 1999. [Sacramento, CA: Department of Health Services], 2001. Available from" URL: http://www.dhs.ca.gov/ ;select "Statistical Resources;" select "Vital Statistics" (accessed May 4, 2001).
3. Ciesielski-Carlucci C, Milliken N, Cohen NH. Determinants of decision making for circumcision. Camb Q Healthc Ethics 5:228-236, 1996.
4. Adler R, Ottaway MS, Gould S. Circumcision: we have heard from the experts; now let's hear from the parents.Pediatrics. 2001 Feb;107(2): E20.
5. O'Brien TR, Calle EE, Poole WK. Incidence of neonatal circumcision in Atlanta, 1985-1986. Southern Med J 1995; 88: 411-415.
6. Binner SL, Mastrobattista JM, Day MC, Swaim LS, Monga M. Effect of parental education on decision-making about neonatal circumcision. South Med J. 2002 Apr;95(4):457-61.
7. Lyon J. Neonatal circumcision in Anchorage 1985-1990. Alaska Med. 1992 Apr-Jun;34(2):94-5.
8. Rickwood AM, Kenny SE, Donnell SC. Towards evidence based circumcision of English boys: survey of trends in practice. BMJ. 2000 Sep 30;321(7264):792-3.
9. Van Howe RS. Variability in penile appearance and penile findings: a prospective study. Br J Urol. 1997 Nov;80(5):776-82.
10. Australian circumcision statistics, from the Health Insurance Commission website http://get.to/gcc and http://guycox.cjb.net

Chapter 14: Religion, History, and Culture
1. Remondino PC. History of Circumcision from the Earliest Times to the Present: Moral and Physical Reasons for its Performance, with a History of Eunuchism, Hermaphrodism, etc., and of the Different Operations Practiced upon the Prepuce. Philadelphia: FA Davis, 1900. (Physicians' and students' ready reference series, no. 11)
2. Harbinson M. Psychosexual Aspects of Circumcision. British Journal of Sexual Medicine. Oct. 1998??

3. Gollaher DL. Circumcision: A History of the World's Most Controversial Surgery. 2000, Basic Books.

4. Rand CS, Emmons CA, Johnson JW.The effect of an educational intervention on the rate of neonatal circumcision. Obstet Gynecol. 1983 Jul;62(1):64-8.

5. Osborn LM, Metcalf TJ, Mariani EM. Hygienic care in uncircumcised infants. Pediatrics. 1981 Mar;67(3):365-7.

6. Herrera AJ, Cochran B, Herrera A, Wallace B. Parental information and circumcision in highly motivated couples with higher education. Pediatrics. 1983 Feb;71(2):233-4.

7. Patton JF. Venereal disease. In: United States Army. Medical Dept. Surgery in World War II: Urology. Washington, DC: Office of the Surgeon General and Center of Military History, United States Army 1987, pp 45-88.

8. Lovell JE, Cox J. Maternal attitudes toward circumcision. J Fam Pract. 1979 Nov;9(5):811-3.

9. Bean GO, Egelhoff C.Neonatal circumcision: when is the decision made? J Fam Pract. 1984 Jun;18(6):883-7.

10. Herrera AJ, Cochran B, Herrera A, Wallace B. Parental information and circumcision in highly motivated couples with higher education. Pediatrics. 1983 Feb;71(2):233-4.

About the Author

Edgar J. Schoen, MD, is a prominent pediatrician who has performed clinical research studies on newborn circumcision which have been published in the leading medical journals. As chairman of the 1989 American Academy of Pediatrics Task Force on Circumcision, he has been involved in developing official medical policies on newborn circumcision. Dr. Schoen has lectured widely at universities and medical centers. For many years he was Chief of Pediatrics and is Senior Consultant in Pediatrics at Kaiser Permanente in Oakland, a large, integrated medical care organization. He is also Clinical Professor of Pediatrics at the University of California, San Francisco.